MENTAL HEALTH CARE

In Settings Where Mental Health Resources Are Limited

An Easy-Reference Guidebook for Healthcare Providers

In Developed and Developing Countries

Pamela Smith, MD

Mental Health Care in Settings Where Mental Health Resources Are Limited:
An Easy-Reference Guidebook for Healthcare Providers
in Developed and Developing Countries

Archway Publishing books may be ordered through booksellers or by contacting:

Archway Publishing
1663 Liberty Drive
Bloomington, IN 47403
www.archwaypublishing.com
1-(888)-242-5904

Because of the dynamic nature of the Internet, any web addresses or links contained in this book may have changed since publication and may no longer be valid. The views expressed in this work are solely those of the author and do not necessarily reflect the views of the publisher, and the publisher hereby disclaims any responsibility for them.

The field guide is not a substitute for comprehensive psychiatry, psychology, or other related mental health texts but is meant to be a concise, quick reference guide providing an outline of core concepts and basic interventions in mental health care. Efforts have been made to confirm the accuracy of the information presented and to describe generally accepted practices. Application of this information in a particular situation remains the responsibility of the practitioner or health care provider.

Certain stock imagery © Thinkstock.
Any people depicted in stock imagery provided by Thinkstock are models, and such images are being used for illustrative purposes only.

ISBN: 978-1-4808-0488-3 (e)
ISBN: 978-1-4808-0487-6 (sc)
ISBN: 978-1-4808-0489-0 (hc)

Library of Congress Control Number: 2014900003

Printed in the United States of America

Archway Publishing rev. date: 1/14/2014

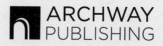

Table of Contents

Table of Contents

Preface & Acknowledgements

In communities where little or no mental health care exists, people with mental conditions are at risk for increased illness, stigma, and abuse. Their fundamental right to mental health & happiness can be compromised. Providing mental health care training to health care workers and raising awareness among individuals within resource-limited communities serves as a significant means not only to improving access to care to individuals but also to preserving human rights. This field guide aims to be a contribution to the broader effort to improve the health, dignity, and quality of life for individuals in resource-limited settings worldwide with mental conditions.

Pamela Smith, MD, completed specialty training in psychiatry at New York – Presbyterian University Hospital of Columbia & Cornell and later served on the faculty of the UCLA Medical School as an assistant clinical professor in psychiatry. She has worked in international humanitarian aid providing mental health support to people living with HIV/AIDS in Uganda, to survivors of the tsunami in Indonesia and Sri Lanka, to survivors of the earthquake in Haiti, and to refugees of the conflict in Darfur, Sudan. Dr. Smith has participated in coordinating projects with organizations and agencies including the AIDS Healthcare Foundation (AHF), International Medical Corps (IMC), World Health Organization (WHO), UNICEF, and United Nations High Commission for Refugees (UNHCR). In addition, she has served on the peer review panel of the United Nations/Inter-Agency Standing Committee Mental Health Task Force developing international guidelines for mental health interventions during emergency disaster relief. Dr. Smith has also provided clinical services (general adult outpatient psychiatry, telepsychiatry) to varied resource-limited communities in urban and rural areas of the United States and has worked for the U.S. Indian Health Services (IHS) supporting the mental health of Native Americans.

A special thanks to Aleksandra Bajic, PharmD for assistance with the medication guide and much gratitude is extended to Whitney A. Relf, PhD, MA (Disabilities Consultant) and Blaire Relf (research assistant) for contributions to the sections on intellectual disability, autism spectrum disorder, ADHD, and Tourette's disorder.

Medical Abbreviations List

bid –twice daily

BP –blood pressure

cap -capsule

CBC –complete blood (cell) count

CNS– central nervous system

DSM -Diagnostic Statistical Manual

dx –diagnosis

EKG– electrocardiogram

EPS-extrapyramidal symptoms

ESR-erythrocyte sedimentation rate

HR– heart rate

ICD– International Classification of Diseases

IM-intramuscular

IV– intravenous

MAOI-monoamine oxidase inhibitor

Meq/L– milliequivalent/liter

mg– milligram

ml– milliliter

MSE– mental status examination

ng– nanogram

NMS– neuroleptic malignant syndrome

po- by mouth

prn -as needed

q –every

qhs– every bedtime

qid– 4 times daily

SNRI– selective norepinephrine reuptake inhibitor

SR - slow release

SSRI-selective serotonin reuptake inhibitor

sx-symptoms

TD– tardive dyskinesia

tid –three times daily

WHO– World Health Organization

XL– extended length

XR– extended release

Introduction

PURPOSE OF THE GUIDE

The guidebook is intended to be a tool for community or hospital-based healthcare providers working in settings where access to mental health resources has been limited or non-existent (e.g. in remotely located, economically impoverished, or nature/human-related disaster-affected communities in developed or developing countries). It is a condensed, easy-reference handbook providing an outline of core concepts and basic interventions in mental health care. The guide is not a substitute for comprehensive psychiatric, psycho-social, or other related mental health texts or training and it is imperative that practitioners or health care workers are responsible in the interpretation and application of information. In addition, differences in cultural beliefs and practices will influence the manner and extent to which the guide is used by individuals in varied regions.

Presented in this guidebook is an allopathic (western) approach to identifying and managing various mental health conditions. The allopathic medical system represents only one method for dealing with mental health issues and other systems of care may have a different relevance or applicability in varied parts of the world.

USING THE GUIDE

How Healthcare Providers Of Varied Disciplines Can Use Different Aspects Of The Guide

Health providers of varied disciplines will find information in the field guide relevant to their practice. In addition, educators can use different aspects of the manual as a source of material for different types and levels of training activity.

All chapters will provide readers with a basic understanding of key topics in the field of mental health. Descriptions of conditions and important issues within the mental health field are written using terminology that can be appreciated by both the professional and the lay person.

The "Medication Guide" section may be especially useful to allopathic physicians and other clinicians such as physician assistants, nurse practitioners, and medical officers (who have the authority to prescribe medication under the supervision of a physician in some countries). In areas using allopathic methods, where nurses, midwives, and social workers are called upon to provide support for people with psychological distress, the counseling interventions, contained in chapters discussing specific mental health conditions, may be particularly useful.

The mental health information contained in this guide useful to varied health care providers (including laypeople, families, and individuals with psychological conditions) is outlined on the following page.

Introduction

MENTAL HEALTH INFORMATION FOUND IN THE GUIDE THAT MAY BE
USEFUL TO HEALTHCARE PROVIDERS OF VARIED DISCIPLINES

Healthcare Provider	General Information & Allopathic Interventions
Health policy-makers & other health administrators; Program Directors	Demographics on mental health care in varied regions of the world
	Integration & collaboration among different health systems
	Mental health duties for primary care providers & mental health service organization and design
Mental Health Trainers; Educators	Mental health training curricula for primary care providers of varied disciplines
Physicians;	Signs and treatment of major mental health conditions; maternal & child mental health
Medical Officers; Physician Assistants, Nurse Practitioners;	How to prescribe psychotropic medication and manage side effects
	Counseling techniques
Pharmacists	Medication therapy for mental health conditions
Nurses; Midwives	Signs and treatment of major mental health conditions
	Maternal & child mental health
	How to administer psychotropic medication & recognize side effects
	Counseling techniques for individuals and groups
Social Workers	Signs of major mental health conditions
	Counseling techniques for individuals and groups; How to provide community education & help communities organize psychosocial activities
Community Mental Health Workers/ Aides	Basic signs of mental distress; support for individuals & groups; How to provide community education & help communities organize psychosocial activities

PART I: MENTAL HEALTH WORLDWIDE

The World Health Organization (WHO) has defined mental health as a "state of well-being in which every individual realizes his or her own potential, can cope with the normal stresses of life, can work productively and fruitfully, and is able to make a contribution to her or his community."

Global mental health refers to the international perspective on varied aspects of mental health and has been defined as "the area of study, research and practice that places a priority on improving mental health and achieving equity in mental health for all people worldwide" (Koplan et al, 2009). Neuropsychiatric disorders contribute to approximately 13% of the global burden of disease and create (to varying degrees among countries) burden in every country in the world.

Assessments of mental health resources worldwide are done with the aim of shedding light on the most recent global view of resources available to prevent neuropsychiatric disorders, provide intervention, and protect human rights. WHO reports of mental health worldwide have examined resources with regard to geographic region and economic status. Categorizing countries into regions is one way to organize the huge volume of information about mental health structures and services throughout the world. In addition, looking at regions may be useful from an economic perspective. It has been established that many nations have no or very limited mental health programming and need to utilize the support of other countries to develop a system of care. Being in a region where a high percentage of neighboring countries have resources can be useful for a country in the same area that has limitations. In addition, using the resources of a nation nearby may be less expensive and a faster process than relying on resources from a far distance.

11

I: Mental Health Worldwide

An examination from the economic perspective allows the identification of specific types of mental health issues prevalent in countries with different income levels. This information can potentially guide the planning of mental health policies, legislation, programs and services. The information may also be useful to funding agencies providing financial support to countries that want to develop resources.

Limitations of Global Studies & Reports

Trying to understand the status of mental health care in countries throughout the world has been a challenging process. Existing reports and studies have taken the best measures possible to be scientific and accurate in collecting, analyzing, and placing in perspective results of data. Nevertheless, these studies are not without their limitations.

With regard to a discussion of mental health care by global region, data may be limited by the way regions have been categorized. In a report on global mental health (WHO, 2005) "regions" are not necessarily divided precisely or purely by global or physical location (i.e. a "region" may include countries that are not physically located on the same continent). In some cases, the "regional" similarity appears to be related to historical, cultural, or economic factors that may link and make a group of countries comparable for analysis.

Other limitations include an inability to obtain information from all countries on all variables, variations in how different countries define mental health concepts, and variations from country to country in sources of information.

I: Mental Health Worldwide

Information presented in this section comes from reports and studies that have inherent limitations, therefore specific conclusions and summary statements will have limitations as well. Data from the WHO is particularly highlighted. One reviewing this information should continue to follow subsequent studies, reports, and related literature from varied sources to gain a full and accurate perspective of global mental health care.

Recent Data

Results of a recent assessment of 184 of 196 World Health Organization (WHO) member states (representing 95% of WHO member states and 98% of the world's population) have indicated that there is a growing burden of neuropsychiatric disease and that mental health resources remain insufficient (WHO 2011). The burden of disease is much greater in low income countries compared to high income countries. However, the number of beds in mental hospitals is reduced in the majority of countries which may be an indication of a shift from institutional care to community-based care.

In the WHO 2011 report, geographic regions were classified as Africa (AFR), the Americas (AMR), Eastern Mediterranean (EMR), Europe (EUR), South/South-East Asia (SEAR), and the Western Pacific (WPR) and income levels were described in terms of high (gross national per capita income of US$ 12, 276 or more), upper-middle (US$ 12,275 – $3,976), lower-middle (US$ 3975 - $1006), and low (US$ 1005 or less). A summary of key findings is provided in the next section.

I: Mental Health Worldwide

Indicators of Global Mental Health (WHO, 2011)

1) Governance
2) Financing
3) Mental health care delivery of services
4) Human resources
5) Medicines for mental & behavioral disorders
6) Information systems.

1) Governance

Mental Health Policy

Data indicates that in about 60% of countries, a dedicated or officially approved mental health policy exists, covering approximately 72% of the world's population. Dedicated mental health policies are more present in EMR, EUR, and SEAR compared to AFR, AMR, and WPR. Data from the World Bank income group also indicates that mental health policies tend to exist in high income countries (77.1%) compared to low income countries (48.7%). Regions with the highest percentage of countries that have recently adopted or updated mental health policies include WPR (87%), EMR (85%), and EUR (84%) while regions with the lowest percentage of countries adopting or revising policies are AFR (56%) and SEAR (57%). The AMR tallied 67% of its countries adopting or updating policies.

I: Mental Health Worldwide

Mental Health Plan

In 72% of the WHO member countries providing data (accounting for 95% of the world's population), a mental health plan (or scheme realizing the objectives of mental health policy) has been outlined. Regions with the greatest percentage of countries with plans include EMR (74%), SEAR (80%) and EUR (81%). Fewer plans were in place in WPR (62%), AMR (66%), and AFR (67%). Regarding income group, wealthier countries had a tendency to have plans compared to countries with low income.

Mental Health Legislation

Worldwide, 59% of people live in a country where dedicated or officially approved mental health legislation exists with legislation present least in AFR (44.4%) and SEAR (40%) and most in AMR (56.3%), EMR (57.9%), EUR (80.8%), and WPR (53.8%). Higher (i.e. high and upper-middle) income countries tended to have legislation present compared to lower (i.e. lower-middle and low) income countries.

2) Financing

The global median mental health expenditures per capita are $1.63 USD. There is a significant difference in median mental health expenditures per capita among income groups, ranging from $0.20 USD in low income countries to $44.84 USD in high income countries. The median percentage of health budget allocated to mental health is highest in the EUR (5.0%), 3.75% in EMR, 1.95% in WPR, 1.53% in AMR, 0.62% in AFR, and 0.44% in SEAR. Regarding income group, the median percentage of health budget allocated to mental health is highest for high income countries (5.1%), 2.38% for upper-middle income countries, 1.90% for lower-middle countries, and lowest or 0.53% for low income countries. Sixty-seven percent (67%) of financial resources world-wide are directed toward mental hospitals /institutions as opposed to community-based facilities (note: only 74 of 184 countries provided responses/data).

3) Mental Care Delivery of Services

The delivery of mental health services has been assessed with regard to a) services provided by primary health care (PHC) clinicians; b) mental health facilities (outpatient, day treatment, general hospital psychiatric ward, community residential, and mental hospital facilities); and c) Aspects of service (length of mental hospital stay, follow up care, psychosocial interventions, and distribution of beds across facilities).

I: Mental Health Worldwide

a) PHC mental health care delivery

A majority of countries allow PHC physicians to prescribe (or continue prescribing) medicines for mental and behavioral disorders either without restrictions (56%) or with some legal restrictions (40%). Restrictions include allowing prescriptions only in emergency settings or in certain categories of medicines. The percentage of respondent countries not allowing any form of prescription by PHC physicians is 3%. Regarding nurses, 71% of countries do not allow them to prescribe (or continue to prescribe), 26% of countries allow prescribing with restrictions, and 3% allow prescribing without restrictions.

b) Mental health facilities

Regarding the number of facilities worldwide, outpatient facilities out number day treatment facilities, mental hospitals, community residential facilities, and psychiatric beds in general hospitals. Outpatient facilities are defined as facilities that focus on the management of mental disorders and related clinical problems on an outpatient basis. A day treatment facility refers to a facility providing care to individuals during the day. A mental hospital is defined as a specialized hospital-based facility that provides inpatient care and long-stay residential services for people with severe mental disorders. A community residential facility is a non-hospital, community-based mental health facility that provides overnight residence for people with mental disorders. The global median number of outpatient facilities is 0.61 (per 100,000 population), 0.05 day treatment facilities, 0.04 mental hospitals, and 0.01 community residential facilities. The global median number of psychiatric beds in general hospitals is 1.4 per 100,000 population.

c) Aspects of mental health service

High income countries tend to have more facilities and higher admission & utilization rates. A majority of people admitted to mental hospitals stay less than one year, however 23 % of those admitted still remain longer than a year.

17

Regarding follow-up care (i.e. home visits to check medications, to monitor signs of relapse, and to assist with rehabilitation), only 32% of countries have a majority of facilities that provide follow-up. Regarding income level 45% of high income countries provide follow-up care at a majority of facilities while 39% of upper-middle income, 29% of lower-middle income, and 7% of low income countries provide follow-up at a majority of facilities.

Regarding psychosocial interventions, only 44% of countries have a majority of countries providing these services. Upper-middle income and high income countries provide more psychosocial care at a majority of facilities(61% and 59% respectively) compared to lower-middle (34%) and low income countries (14%).

The global median rate for all beds in community residential facilities, mental hospitals, and psychiatric wards within general hospitals is 3.2 beds per 100,000 population. Across WHO regions, there is great disparity. That is, the rates in the AFR (0.60), EMR (0.62) and SEAR (0.23) are significantly lower than the global mean, while the rate in EUR countries (7.09) is more than double the world median.

4) Human resources

Worldwide, nurses represent the most common health professional graduate working in the mental health sector (5.15 per 100,000 population). Globally, the next most common health professional graduate working in the mental health sector is the medical doctor (3.38 per 100,000 population). Regarding psychiatrists, the median rate ranges from 0.05 per 100,000 population in AFR to 8.59 per 100,000 population in EUR. Regarding other health personnel working in the mental health sector, the median rate of other medical doctors ranges from 0.06 (AFR) to 1.14 (EUR) per 100,000 and for nurses ranges from 0.61 (AFR) to 21.93 (EUR) per 100,000. The median rate of psychologists ranges from 0 (WPR) to 2.58 (EUR) per 100,000; social workers from 0 (WPR) to 1.12 (EUR) per 100,000; occupational therapists from 0 (SEAR and WPR) to 0.57 (EUR) per 100,000; and other health workers from

0.04 (SEAR) to 17.21 (EUR) per 100,000.

With regard to income group, there is significant disparity in the number of doctors, nurses, and psychologists working in the mental health sector. For psychologists, the median rate of these clinicians working in the mental health sector is over 180 times greater in high income compared to low income countries. In high income countries, the median rate of psychiatrists is 8.59 compared to 0.05 in low income countries.

Worldwide, 2.8% of training for doctors is focused on psychiatry and mental health related topics. Variability across regions exists ranging from 2.2% in AMR to 4.0% in SEAR. For nurses, 3.3% of training is focused on psychiatry and mental health-related topics with moderate variability among regions ranging from 2.0% in SEAR and 4.0% in AFR

5) Medicines for mental & behavioral disorders

Worldwide, the median expenditure per person per year on medicines for mental and behavioral disorders has been estimated to be about $7 ($6.81) USD. However, the actual expenditure is likely to be lower, as fewer than 30% of countries involved in the recent WHO survey reported data, with those responding being disproportionately from high income countries.

6) Information systems

According to the WHO 2011 report, mental health data is collected for individuals receiving treatment from mental hospitals, general medical hospitals, day treatment and outpatient facilities. Less data tends to be collected from primary care and community residential facilities.

PART II. MENTAL HEALTH CAPACITY BUILDING:

**Increasing Access to Care Through Integration
& Collaboration**

INTEGRATING MENTAL HEALTH CARE INTO EXISTING
HEALTH FACILITIES

Integrating mental health care into existing community facilities
can be an effective and efficient way to deliver mental health services to a large number of people living in areas with limited resources.

The integration process involves **training** existing primary healthcare practitioners based in the community and has been utilized in
western (allopathic) health systems. General practitioners and
healthcare workers are trained to make basic mental health assessments, to provide basic therapeutic interventions, and to refer to
more specialized interventions (if available) individuals who have
more serious psychiatric symptoms.

The integration process may also involve working with government agencies and other institutions to develop mental health policies, to promote deinstitutionalization and provision of community
-based acute and continuing care (for those with the most serious
and disabling conditions), and to incorporate mental health training
programs into medical, nursing, and graduate schools.

II. Mental Health Capacity Building

Telepsychiatry

Telepsychiatry refers to the use of communications and information technologies for training and, in some cases, directly delivering mental health care. It has been especially beneficial for populations living in isolated communities and remote regions. Through video-conferencing (one form of technology) general practitioners in areas with limited or no access to mental health services can gain access to a mental health specialist located in a different region for ongoing consultations and supervision. In addition, mental health training programs that utilize telepsychiatry have the potential to reduce costs while maintaining an efficient and effective means for providing technical advice and information.

RECOMMENDATIONS FOR MENTAL HEALTH TRAINING CURRICULA & DUTIES FOR VARIED HEALTHCARE PERSONNEL

Suggested curricula and duties for varied primary care providers are outlined in the tables on the following pages. In addition, guidelines on how to teach primary healthcare staff to provide mental health care are offered in the pages to follow.

II. Mental Health Capacity Building

Physicians, Medical Officers, Physician Assistants, Nurse Practitioners

Suggested Mental Health Curriculum	Suggested Duties

A. The Psychiatric History & Mental Status Exam
 	
B. Symptoms, Diagnosis & Treatment of:
 	
1. Schizophrenia & Other Psychotic Conditions
 	
2. Mood Disorders
 	
3. Anxiety Disorders
 	
4. Somatic Symptom Disorder & Psychological Factors Affecting Other Medical Conditions
 	
5. Delirium (Neuro-cognitive disorders)
 	
6. Dementia (Neuro-cognitive disorders)
 	
7. Alcohol & Drug Use Disorders
 	
8. Epilepsy/Seizures Disorders
 	
9. Maternal Mental Health; Neuro-developmental Disorders and Common Psychiatric & Behavioral Conditions in Children & Adolescents
 	
10. Loss & Bereavement
 	
11. Psychiatric Emergencies (suicide/ agitation)
 	
C. Other Issues:
 	
  1. Institutionalization
 	
  2. Mental Health Care in Disaster Relief
 	
  3. Stigma and discrimination & legal and ethical issues in the mental health setting
	a) Perform psychiatric history and mental status examination; formulate diagnoses and treatment plans
	
	b) Prescribe psychotropic medication and manage side effects
	
	c) Provide counseling directly or provide referral to staff implementing counseling

II. Mental Health Capacity Building

Nurses & Midwives

Suggested Mental Health Curriculum	Suggested Duties
A. The Psychiatric History & Mental Status Exam	

B. Symptoms, Diagnosis & Treatment of:
 	
  1. Schizophrenia & Other Psychotic Conditions
 	
  2. Mood Disorders
 	
  3. Anxiety Disorders
 	
  4. Somatic Symptom Disorder & Psychological Factors Affecting Other Medical Conditions
 	
  5. Delirium (Neuro-cognitive disorders)
 	
  6. Dementia (Neuro-cognitive disorders)
 	
  7. Alcohol & Drug Use Disorders
 	
  8. Epilepsy/Seizure Disorders
 	
  9. Maternal Mental Health; Neuro-developmental Disorders and Common Psychiatric & Behavioral Conditions in Children & Adolescents
 	
  10. Loss & Bereavement
 	
  11. Psychiatric Emergencies (suicide/ agitation)
	a) Perform mental health evaluations; child development assessments (in some countries midwives may be focused on this activity); refer to physician for medications if indicated
	
	b) Administer medications prescribed by physicians *(*nurses & midwives in some countries also prescribe under physician supervision)*
	
	c) Recognize medication side effects and refer to the physician for treatment

C. Other issues:
 	
  1. Community Mental Health Nursing
 	
  2. Institutionalization
 	
  3. Mental Health Care in Disaster Relief
 	
  4. Stigma and discrimination & legal and ethical issues in the mental health setting
 	
  5. Mental health promotion, psycho-education, and advocacy
	d) Implement counseling techniques directly or refer to staff who implement counseling

II. Mental Health Capacity Building

Social Workers

Suggested Mental Health Curriculum	Suggested Duties
A. The Psychiatric History & Mental Status Exam	
B. Symptoms, Diagnosis & Treatment of:	a) Provide guidance regarding basic needs (food, shelter, safety, education, access to healthcare, etc…)
1. Schizophrenia & Other Psychotic Conditions	
2. Mood Disorders	
3. Anxiety Disorders	b) Refer individuals in need to mental health evaluation (in some countries social workers perform evaluations)
4. Somatic Symptom Disorder & Psychological Factors Affecting Other Medical Conditions	
5. Delirium (Neuro-cognitive disorders)	c) Implement counseling (in some countries social workers implement individual, family, & group counseling)
6. Dementia (Neuro-cognitive disorders)	
7. Alcohol & Drug Use Disorders	
8. Epilepsy/Seizure Disorders	d) Implement community education (focused on stigma; maintaining mental wellness; and recognition of signs of psychological distress)
9. Maternal Mental Health; Neuro-developmental Disorders and Common Psychiatric & Behavioral Conditions in Children & Adolescents	
10. Loss & Bereavement	e) Assist communities in organizing psychosocial activities
11. Psychiatric Emergencies (suicide/ agitation)	
C. Other issues:	
1. Institutionalization	
2. Mental Health Care in Disaster Relief	
3. Stigma and discrimination & legal and ethical issues in the mental health setting	
4. Mental health promotion, education, and advocacy	

II. Mental Health Capacity Building

Community Mental Health Workers/Aides

Suggested Mental Health Curriculum	Suggested Duties
A. Basic Signs & Symptoms of:	
1. Schizophrenia & Other Psychotic Conditions	
2. Mood Disorders	a) Identify and refer individuals in need to mental health evaluations
3. Anxiety Disorders	
4. Somatic Symptom Disorder & Psychological Factors Affecting Other Medical Conditions	
5. Delirium (Neuro-cognitive disorders)	b) Provide individual, family, & group psychological support
6. Dementia (Neuro-cognitive disorders)	
7. Alcohol & Drug Use Disorders	c) Implement community education (focused on stigma; maintaining mental wellness; and recognition of signs of psychological distress)
8. Epilepsy/Seizure disorders	
9. Maternal Mental Health; Neuro-developmenal Disorders and Common Psychiatric & Behavioral Conditions in Children & Adolescents	
10. Loss & Bereavement	
11. Psychiatric Emergencies (suicide; agitation)	
B. Basic Types of Support Available in the Community	d) Assist communities in organizing psychosocial activities
C. How to Refer Individuals in the Community to Evaluation and Support	
D. Basic Information on:	
1. Mental Health Care in Disaster Relief	
2. Institutionalization	
3. Stigma and discrimination & legal and ethical issues in the mental health setting	
4. Mental health promotion, psycho-education, and advocacy	

II. Mental Health Capacity Building

GUIDELINES FOR TEACHING PRIMARY HEALTHCARE
STAFF TO PROVIDE MENTAL HEALTH CARE

One approach to training primary healthcare staff to provide mental health care involves a) establishing learning goals and objectives that are relevant and applicable to the existing practices of the primary care staff; b) developing theoretical mental health presentations and practical on-the-job supervision sessions that are effective and convenient; and c) utilizing comprehensive evaluations to monitor and further enhance learning. It is important that those teaching have the appropriate level of education or experience in their areas of instruction and that trainees have a basic level of understanding that will allow them to comprehend the instruction.

A) Establishing Learning Goals & Objectives – What is the information trainees are expected to learn?

Objectives may be defined as the learning needed to reach a particular goal. Trainers must decide on the desired goal of their training sessions and then develop clear objectives that will lead to the goal.

Goals and objectives need to be relevant or directly applicable to the real situations staff face in their primary care settings.

Example: A goal of a mental health training course for a group of primary care doctors may be that they learn to provide an effective treatment for an individual with a particular mental health condition. Objectives toward this goal may include their a) learning to take a psychiatric history; b) learning the varied signs and symptoms of varied mental health conditions; and c) learning the varied types of therapies to manage conditions. A number of objectives may be involved in achieving an overall goal.

II. Mental Health Capacity Building

B) Theoretical Presentations & On-the Job Supervision

Lecture presentations

Theoretical information may be presented in many forms. A lecture format that is interactive (i.e. involves audience participation) and offers a clear outline can be effective. However, lengthy or numerous lectures should be minimized for primary care staff who may be overwhelmed already with several tasks and responsibilities. Staff participating in training sessions will absorb more information if it is presented in a manner that is concise and relates directly to their existing work activities.

It can be helpful to consider the Who, What/Why, Where, and How when outlining a lecture:

1) Who are you presenting to?

a) Understand who your audience is; know their level of education, experience or understanding in general;

b) Always treat the audience respectfully and allow questions; provide clear explanations;

c) Take time to put an audience and yourself at ease by having some informal interaction before getting into the core presentation (e.g. use opening joke, story or "ice-breaker" activity).

2) <u>What</u> information or skills do you need them to understand and <u>Why</u> is this information important for them to know?

a) Start with a welcome and introduction (and informal interaction);

b) Reiterate why it is important that they have attended;

c) Provide an outline of the session that states topics to be discussed and a general time frame for the discussion;

d) Make clear what they can expect from the session (desired outcome and objectives) and why it is important for them to attain this information;

e) Start with a broad outline of the information and then get more specific;

f) Conclude with a summary of the key points of the discussion.

3) <u>Where</u> will you be presenting the information?

a)Take time to prepare your space so that it is conducive to effective learning (Is there enough space for all participants to see and hear you? Are there electrical outlets in the room? Is there an adequate setting for breaks?; Are toilets nearby? etc...).

4) Specifically <u>How</u> will I present the information (what types of materials or aids will be useful in presenting the information)?

a) What aids are available and feasible to use (chalkboard or white-board? projectors?; flip charts?; microphones? Is there electricity or a generator to power electronic aides? Etc...);

b) Are take-home materials used (books, handouts, brochures, etc...).

On-the-job supervision

Theoretical information must be practically applied to real situations faced by the primary care staff. Having a knowledgeable supervisor teach and monitor as a trainee works directly with patients will reinforce that trainee's learning and understanding of the theoretical concepts. Clients should be made aware of the role of the supervisor prior to sessions and should be reassured that information will not be used inappropriately.

C) Evaluation Of Teaching

Evaluations of the trainees and trainers (and training programs) are indicators of whether or not teaching has been effective and learning has been achieved. Evaluations are also useful in monitoring progress and providing feedback and guidance on how to enhance the instruction and learning process. Outlined in the box on the following page are elements that may be included in evaluations.

II. Mental Health Capacity Building

Elements of Training Evaluations

The following information can be useful in monitoring and determining the effectiveness of trainings:

1) Trainee evaluation

        Trainee name (use ID numbers for confidentiality)

        Trainee level of education/experience in MH care

        Dates of participation and completion of coursework

        list of all sessions/courses completed

        list of courses repeated

        theoretical & practical examination scores

        theoretical & practical re-examination scores

2) Trainer & program/course/session evaluation

        trainee survey evaluating quality of teaching, coursework, and examinations (was trainer an effective speaker/communicator; were topics clear; were teaching aids adequate; did exam questions reflect material presented, etc…)

3) Program/course/session evaluation

        total trainee enrollment

        number of trainees with successful completion of the program

        trainee attrition (number of drop-outs before completion of the program)

        number of trainees requiring repetition of coursework/re-examination

        progress/clinical outcome (condition of patients treated by trainees at the start of treatment compared to their condition at the end of treatment)

        patient/community survey evaluating services provided by trainees

II. Mental Health Capacity Building

HOW TO DEVELOP COLLABORATIONS

Cultures and societies throughout the world and throughout time have found ways to describe and manage human emotions and behavior. Some societies have created organized systems of mental health care while others have adopted different approaches. Collaboration implies a coexistence among systems and approaches with each contributing its own unique methods for managing the health of individuals. The advantage of a health care system that utilizes collaboration is that varied options for care become available, increasing the potential for effective outcomes.

<u>Ways that practitioners from different health systems develop collaborations</u>

a) Invitations to consultations;

b) Cross-referral - For example, some problems may potentially be better treated by one form of medicine compared to another (e.g. stress, anxiety, bereavement, conversion reactions, and existential distress may be managed with significant effect by non-allopathic practitioners, while allopathic practitioners may be have more effective treatments for severe mental disorders and epilepsy);

c) Joint assessments;

d) Joint training sessions;

e) Joint clinics;

f) Shared care (e.g. non-allopathic practitioners may be prepared to learn how to monitor psychotic patients on long-term allopathic medication and to provide places for patients to stay while receiving allopathic treatments).

II. Mental Health Capacity Building

Advantages of collaboration

a) Increased understanding of the way emotional distress and psychiatric illness is expressed and addressed and a more comprehensive picture of the type and level of distress in the affected population;

b) Improved referral systems;

c) Continuing relationship with healers of varied types to whom many people turn for help;

d) Increased understanding of community members' spiritual, psychological and social worlds;

e) Greater acceptance of new services by community members;

f) Identifying opportunities for potential collaborative efforts in healing and thus increasing the number of potentially effective treatments available to the population;

g) Establishing services that may be more culturally appropriate;

h) The potential opportunity to monitor and address any human rights abuses occurring within different systems of care.

Activities Prior to Collaboration

Before pursuing collaboration in an unfamiliar setting, the healthcare provider should first develop (as best as possible) an understanding of the national policies and attitudes regarding various types of practitioners. For example, some governments discourage or ban health care providers from collaborating with traditional healers. Other governments encourage collaboration and have special departments engaged in the formal training of healers, as well as in research and evaluation of traditional medicine.

II. Mental Health Capacity Building

Organizing Collaborations

To facilitate collaboration, the healthcare provider should make an assessment of the other systems of care present in the community. This may be difficult for providers who are outsiders to the community. Being respectful and establishing trust with members of the community is very important. Outlined below are suggestions on how to obtain information about other systems.

a) Contact local community members who are a diverse sample of the community if possible (i.e. speak to women, men, elderly/adolescent individuals, members of different ethnicities, etc…). Ask them where they seek help for mental health difficulties and whom they use for emotional support.

b) Ask primary health care providers and midwives what systems exist, including pharmacies.

c) Ask the people encountered in the health facilities how they perceive their problems, and who else they see or have seen previously for assistance.

d) Contact local religious leaders and ask whether they provide supportive or healing services and who else in the community does so.

e) Use the help of community representatives or providers to organize a meeting with the local practitioners.

f) Remember that more than one system of care may exist, and that practitioners in one system may not acknowledge or discuss others.

g) Be aware that within a community, local practitioners may compete over patients or be in conflict over the appropriate approach.

II. Mental Health Capacity Building

It is important next to establish a rapport and ongoing dialogue with the practitioners. Encouraging and actively organizing forums for information-sharing and cross-training is important. A variety of practitioners should play a role in the trainings and discussions about practical administrative issues, such as creating a cross- referral process should be included on agendas. After a series of effective trainings has occurred, consider organizing specific collaborative services where needed (if possible).

A Caution Regarding Some Healing Practices

It should be noted that some healing practices may be harmful, since they include beatings, prolonged fasting, cutting, prolonged physical restraint or expulsion of 'witches' from the community. The challenge in such cases is to find constructive ways of addressing harmful practices, as far as is realistic. Before supporting or collaborating with any healing practice, it is essential to determine what those practices include and whether they are potentially beneficial, neutral, or harmful. Sometimes maintaining a respectful distance is the best option, rather than seeking collaboration.

PART III. MENTAL HEALTH CONDITIONS & ISSUES:

Identification and Interventions

OVERVIEW

The allopathic (western) medical system represents one approach to dealing with mental health issues and managing mental health conditions. Allopathic mental health care may be described as a system of care in which staff has been trained in medical science, behavioral science, formal psychotherapy and provides services in inpatient hospitals, outpatient clinics, and other community facilities. This system of care is one form of support that is used today, commonly in high-income societies. Non-allopathic types of care may include traditional, indigenous, complementary, alternative, informal, and local medicine and in some countries are utilized as a primary or complementary means of care. These systems may involve the use of animal or mineral based medicines, religious or spiritual interventions, and manual techniques, either singularly or in combination.

Presented in this part of the guidebook is an allopathic approach to managing various mental health conditions. Basic theoretical concepts, counseling interventions, and medication therapies are described.

HOW TO IDENTIFY PSYCHOLOGICAL SYMPTOMS

Descriptions of mental health and illness

Someone with a "healthy mind" has clear thoughts, the ability to solve the problems of daily life, enjoys good relationships with friends, family, and work colleagues, is spiritually at ease, and can bring happiness to others (V.Patel 2002).

Mental illness can be defined as any illness experienced by a person which affects their emotions, thoughts or behavior, is out of keeping with their cultural beliefs and personality, and produces a negative effect on their lives or the lives of their families. Symptoms of illness can appear in the form of persistent changes in mood, perception of reality, or capacity to organize or maintain thoughts. Such changes will interfere with the person's usual beliefs, personality or social function.

The psychiatric history & mental status examination (MSE) are tools used to identify psychological distress and symptoms of illness. Information and observations obtained can be used to guide the healthcare provider's impressions and therapeutic interventions.

III. Conditions & Issues: How to Identify Symptoms

The Psychiatric History

Psychological distress and mental illness may be influenced by past and present experiences and circumstances. A psychiatric history is a description of the habits, activities, relationships, and physical conditions that have shaped the way one feels, thinks, and behaves. The psychiatric history is obtained by interviewing the individual or asking a series of questions associated with their psychological function. Outlined below are the standard elements of the psychiatric history.

Elements of the Psychiatric History

1)   Identifying data – name, age, race, sex.

2)   Chief complaint – a concise statement of the patient's psychiatric problem in his or her own words.

3)   History of present illness – current circumstances in which current psychiatric symptoms have occurred.

4)   Previous psychiatric history – any prior psychiatric symptoms, treatment (therapy or medication); prior psychiatric hospitalizations.

5)   Medical history – history of significant medical conditions, treatments/surgeries; current medications; history of allergies to medications or other agents; history of head injuries; seizures; loss of consciousness or other neurological disorders.

6)   Family psychiatric history – any blood relatives with history of psychiatric symptoms, treatment, or psychiatric hospitalizations.

7)   History of alcohol or drug abuse or dependence – length or period of abuse/dependence; date and amount of last use; history of drug treatment or rehabilitation programs.

8)   Social history – place of birth; description of family members; marital status; education obtained; occupations past and present.

The Mental Status Examination

The purpose of the MSE is to assess the individual's current emotional state and capacity for mental function. The mental status examination is an organized systematic framework for noting observations that are made while interviewing individuals. In general, it involves categorizing observations in terms of behavior and appearance; thought, feelings, judgment, insight, and other functions such as memory and concentration.

41

III. Conditions & Issues: How to Identify Symptoms

Elements of the Mental Status Examination (MSE)

1) General Appearance – e.g. gait; grooming; posture.

2) Motoric behavior (i.e. physical movements)–e.g. physical agitation or retardation; tremors; anxiety.

3) Speech – e.g. slow; rapid; loud; soft/inaudible; stuttering; slurring; paucity; over-inclusive.

4) Attitude –e.g. cooperative; irritable; angry; aggressive; defensive; guarded; apathetic.

5) Mood – e.g. sad; happy; irritable; angry; elevated or expansive.

6) Affect or facial expression – e.g. congruent or incongruent with mood; flat; blunted; fluctuating.

7) Thought content – e.g. delusions (persistent belief that is inconsistent with reality), paranoia; suicidal or homicidal thoughts.

8) Thought processing – e.g. logical/illogical; repetitive; disjointed; tendency to go on tangent; concrete. Decelerated; slowed; rapid succession of ideas.

9) Perception – e.g. auditory, visual, tactile, or olfactory hallucinations.

10) Judgment – e.g. ability to understand relationships between facts and to draw appropriate conclusions.

11) Insight – e.g. is the patient able or willing to understand his or her condition?

12) Cognition

    a) level of consciousness – e.g. alert; cloudy; confused.

    b) orientation - i.e. to self, place, date, time.

    c) memory – i.e. long-term (events of the past such as place of birth; date of marriage or graduations); recent (events of yesterday or last week); short-term (test recall of 3 items after a period of 5 minutes).

    d) concentration or attention (serial 7 test – start at 100 and count backwards by 7).

    e) executive function or ability to reason – test using abstraction tasks (e.g. ask how are an apple and banana similar? Ask individual to interpret a proverb appropriate to culture); test naming or word finding skill (e.g. can the individual name different parts of a watch/time-piece).

    f) visual-motor coordination, in basic terms, may be defined as the brain's ability to coordinate information perceived by a sensory organ (the eyes) with complex motor functions (such as writing). Visual-motor coordination is tested by asking the individual to draw an object or figure visualized. For example, draw a circle that is connected to a rectangle and ask the individual to copy the figure. An inability to copy the figure accurately may be an indication of conditions such as brain damage due to medical disease or drug abuse (e.g. Alzheimer's disease; alcohol dementia;), schizophrenia, or mental retardation.

43

PSYCHOTIC CONDITIONS:

Schizophrenia & Other Psychotic Conditions

The term "psychosis" has been used to describe individuals who misinterpret reality or experience and express distortions (out of the realm of reality) in perception, thought, and feeling. Distortions may lead to disruption in function with family, friends at school, or at work. Some psychotic conditions may run in families and their specific causes are not fully understood while other psychotic conditions are due to medical conditions or substances affecting the mental state.

Schizophrenia

Schizophrenia is a chronic disorder that may be characterized by a decline in motivation, socialization and function, diminished emotional expression, disorganized or abnormal motor behavior (i.e. physical movement) and distorted sense of reality (with disturbances in perception and/or the expression of thought). Worldwide prevalence estimates have ranged between 0.5% and 1%. Theories regarding the cause have been proposed and have included a genetic, biological, psychosocial, and infectious basis for the disease. Schizophrenia has been described in many cultures.

Signs/Characteristics of Schizophrenia

* Decline in level of function and ability to socialize (this can be expressed as withdrawal, detachment or isolation from others; this may also be expressed as aggression).

* Thoughts are expressed in an impaired or illogical manner (i.e. incoherence; one may appear to have long pauses, a "blank" or a lapse in thought; one may easily or repeatedly lose the point in conversation; thoughts are disjointed with the association between thoughts being lost).

* Delusional thought (thoughts that are inconsistent with reality and persistently maintained).

* Impaired perception (hallucinations – auditory hallucinations or hearing people or things that are not physically present are the most common in schizophrenia; visual hallucinations or hallucinations of taste, touch, and smell may occur but are less common).

* Diminished or incongruent emotional expressions (appearing expressionless; crying easily over things that are not typically sad); abnormal physical movement (catatonia).

* Altered motivation (ambivalence about doing activities or complete loss of motivation for activities).

* Symptoms persist (for at least 6 months) and are not due to a medical condition or substance abuse.

Other Psychotic Conditions (DSM V/ US classification system)

Aside from schizophrenia, psychosis may occur due to other conditions including delusional disorder (delusion is the prominent symptom); schizophreniform (schizophrenia-like symptoms for < 6 months); schizo-affective disorder (both mood and psychotic symptoms are prominent); brief psychosis (psychotic symptoms<1 month); post partum psychosis (psychotic symptoms after giving birth); and psychosis secondary to psychoactive substances or medical conditions.

Counseling Interventions For Schizophrenia & Other Psychotic Conditions

1. Outline a weekly schedule with the individual. A structured routine helps one to know what to do and expect - this can reduce the stress and anxiety that can precipitate symptoms. Clearly list the core activities of daily living (showering, shaving, dressing, supply shopping, food preparation, cleaning) so that basic self-care skills are maintained. Include chores so that a sense of responsibility is maintained. Include pleasure activities. Be sure there is a good balance between indoor and outdoor activities. Also be sure to incorporate activities that involve social interaction.

2. Reward constructive actions. Determine the items or situations that the patient values and reward him/her with them when appropriate behavior is displayed (e.g. offer a valued reward for having completed all chores and activities of daily living adequately).

3. Help the individual identify situations that cause stress or anxiety as these can be triggers for a relapse of illness. Help the individual limit involvement in these situations. If the situation is unavoidable, help the individual think in advance about what may occur and how he/she will respond.

4. Emphasize medication compliance. Discuss with the doctor medication options and regimens that will make taking pills easy.

5. Ask the health provider to explain the kind of side effects that might be expected and what to do about them.

6. Emphasize keeping track of appointments. Missed appointments and doses of medicine can put the patient at risk for a return of illness.

7. Educate family or caretakers. Educate that agitation or odd behavior are symptoms of schizophrenia and are not intentional. Relapse is possible and should be anticipated. Review the signs and symptoms of schizophrenia.

Medication Therapy

See the "Medication Guide" section of the manual for details on medication therapy.

MOOD –RELATED CONDITIONS:

Major Depression & Bipolar Disorder

Major Depression

Depression has been generally described as a decline in mood that persists for an extended period, represents a decrease from a previous level of function, and causes some impairment in function. Depression contributes significantly to the global burden of disease affecting an estimated 350 million people worldwide. According to the World Mental Health Survey (conducted in 17 countries) approximately 1 in 20 people on average reported an episode of depression in the previous year. In many cultures depression is expressed commonly as somatic or physical complaints (e.g. fatigue, generalized pain, digestive problems, headache). Psychotic symptoms may also occur. Other signs and characteristics of depression are outlined below.

Signs & Characteristics

- Persistent depressed mood and loss of pleasure in activities that normally give pleasure;

- weight loss or gain;

- insomnia (i.e. too little sleep) or hypersomnia (i.e. too much sleep);

- psychomotor agitation (i.e. agitated movement) or retardation (i.e. slowed movement); energy loss;

- feelings of worthlessness or guilt;

- poor concentration or memory; indecisiveness;

- hopelessness or suicidal thoughts with the intention to act or with specific plans made;

49

- symptoms are not due to a medical condition or substance capable of influencing the central nervous system.

Studies have indicated that biological, genetic, and psychosocial factors play a role in depression. Biological factors include disturbances in neurotransmitters (molecules mediating communication between brain cells), abnormal immune system function, and abnormal regulation of hormones. Genetic causes have been implicated through studies of patterns of illness in families (e.g. first degree relatives, twins) and studies of genetic material. Psychosocial factors (life events and environmental stressors) have been suggested as an influence as well. Depression may be diagnosed through psychiatric history, mental status examination and eliminating other causes with laboratory or other diagnostic tests. Depression is treated with counseling interventions and, in severe cases, medication.

Counseling Interventions for Depression

If symptoms are persistent and severe, refer to a crisis center/doctor/hospital for further evaluation, diagnosis, & treatment.

Offer support: emphasize that there is no shame in feeling depressed; help the individual identify others who can serve as a support (family, friends); help him/her identify & focus on personal strengths and the positives in a challenging situation; help him/her identify & focus on what they can control; ask about hopeless and suicidal feelings and the intent to act on these feelings.

Medication Therapy

See the "Medication Guide" section of the manual for details on medication therapy.

Bipolar Disorder

Bipolar disorder is a type of mood disorder characterized by distinct phases of sustained depression and/or distinct periods of a mood which is persistent and abnormally elevated, expansive , or irritable. Psychosis may be present also in either phase. According to research analyzing World Health Organization (WHO) mental health survey data, the prevalence rates for bipolar spectrum disorder (BPS) worldwide vary, but illness severity and patterns of co-morbidity are similar.

The table below outlines important features of the most severe form of bipolar disorder, bipolar type I disorder.

Signs & Characteristics

DISOR-DER	ETIOLOGY (cause)	SYMPTOMS	DIAGNOSIS
Bipolar I	- Evidence for Genetics as a factor - Biological factors - Environmental factors	*Manic Phase*: Elevated/irritable mood; excessive energy or agitation; elevated esteem or grandiosity; rapid thoughts; decreased need for sleep; excessive or pressured speech; distractibility; impulsive, potentially harmful behavior *Depressive Phase:* depressive symptoms satisfy criteria for a full major depressive episode (SEE DEPRESSION SECTION OF THIS CHAPTER FOR SPECIFIC SYMPTOMS)	Symptoms are identified through mental status examination (MSE); Rule out substance and medical causes via diagnostic tests if available (i.e. toxicology screens, thyroid function tests, chemistries, CBC, brain imaging)

51

Other Types of Bipolar Disorders

1) Bipolar II – presence of at least one major depressive
   episode and one hypomanic (i.e. less severely manic)
   episode. No manic episode has occurred. The criteria
   for a hypomanic episode is the same as for a manic
   episode except that in a hypomanic episode the symptoms do not cause significant impairment in social or
   occupational function. Psychosis may occur with this
   condition.

2) Substance/Medication induced Bipolar Disorder - persistent and prominent elevated, expansive, or irritable
   mood (with or without depressive symptoms) that occurs in the context of using a substance or medication
   which can cause bipolar symptoms. The disturbance
   causes significant distress or impaired function. The
   disturbance does not occur during a period of delirium.

Counseling interventions for Mania/Bipolar Disorder

1. Educate the family/caretakers. Educate the family and patient that agitation, mood fluctuation, and impulsivity are common symptoms of bipolar disorder and are not intentional. Relapse is possible and should be anticipated. Review with them the signs and symptoms of bipolar disorder. Emphasize the importance of medication compliance.

2. Emphasize medication compliance. Discuss with the doctor medication options and regimens that will make taking pills easy (e.g. use of pill organizer boxes; explore whether once a day dosing is appropriate and possible).

3. Reward constructive actions. Determine the items or situations that the patient values and reward him/her with them when appropriate behavior is displayed (e.g. offer a valued reward for having contained impulsive behaviors).

4. Encourage a routine schedule. Outline a weekly schedule with the individual. A structured routine helps one to know what to do and expect and helps to reduce the stress and anxiety that can precipitate symptoms.

5. Help the individual identify situations that cause stress or anxiety as these can be triggers for a relapse of illness. Help the individual limit involvement in these situations. If a stressful situation is unavoidable, help the patient think in advance about what may occur and how he/she will respond. Breathing and relaxation exercises can reduce anxiety felt in these situations (see chapter on "Anxiety Conditions" for breathing and relaxation exercises).

6. Emphasize keeping track of appointments. Missed appointments can lead to the individual's running out of medication. Missing doses of medicine can put the individual at risk for a return of symptoms and a relapse of illness.

Medication Therapy

See "Medication Guide" section of manual.

III: Conditions & Issues: Anxiety-Related Conditions, OCD, & PTSD

ANXIETY-RELATED CONDITIONS, OBSESSIVE-COMPULSIVE DISORDER (OCD) & POST-TRAUMATIC STRESS DISORDER (PTSD)

Anxiety may be defined as a state of neurological arousal characterized by both physical and psychological signs. Anxiety may be a normal reaction that acts as a signal to the body that aspects of its systems are under stress. Prevalence estimates of anxiety disorders are generally higher in developed countries than in developing countries according to global mental health survey data. The specific neuro-biological mechanisms underlying anxiety are complex and may involve genetic, biological, and psychological factors. Common signs of anxiety are outlined in the table below:

Physical signs	Psychological signs
Headache	Feeling of dread
Muscle tension	Poor concentration
Back pain	Impaired sleep
Abdominal pain	Impaired sexual desire
Tremulousness or "shakiness"	
Fatigue	
Numbness	
Shortness of breath	
Palpitations	
Sweating	
Hyper-vigilant reflexes (easily startled; "jumpy")	

55

III: Conditions & Issues: Anxiety-Related Conditions, OCD, & PTSD

Anxiety "disorders" are considered when the signals triggered by the body produce prolonged physical or psychological discomfort or a pattern and degree of distress that disrupts normal function. An anxiety disorder is considered if no underlying medical illness, substance intoxication (or withdrawal), medication toxicity, or toxicity of other agents can be identified as the cause. Types of anxiety disorders, obsessive-compulsive disorder or OCD, and post-traumatic stress disorder or PTSD (described in western literature/DSM-V) are outlined below.

1. Anxiety-Related Disorders (Anxiety Disorders)

A) Generalized Anxiety Disorder (GAD)

GAD is defined as chronic, constant anxiety that persists throughout the day consistently for at least 1 month.

B) Panic Disorder

Panic disorder involves a sudden, spontaneous onset of overwhelming anxiety symptoms.

C) Agoraphobia

Agoraphobia involves experiencing anxiety and fear in the context of feeling unable to escape in situations such as being in open or enclosed spaces, of being alone outside the home, or of being in a crowd, or using public transportation.

D) Phobia

An irrational fear of a particular object or situation causing anxiety symptoms.

E) Social Phobia/Social Anxiety Disorder

Specific irrational fear/discomfort in social or public situations.

2. Obsessive-Compulsive Disorder (OCD)

The presence of obsessions (i.e. constant intrusive thoughts or urges causing anxiety symptoms) and/or compulsions (i.e. unusual and excessive behaviors or mental acts one is compelled to perform repetitively in order to reduce anxiety to a dreaded situation or event).

3. Post-traumatic Stress Disorder (PTSD) & Acute Stress Disorder

Anxiety occurs in the context of an overwhelming major life stressor. The stressful event is continuously re-experienced (during dreams or wakefulness) causing hyper-arousal and a tendency toward avoidance. If symptoms persist for greater than 1 month PTSD is indicated; if symptoms persist for less than 1 month, acute stress disorder is diagnosed.

III: Conditions & Issues: Anxiety-Related Conditions, OCD, & PTSD

Counseling Interventions: Exercises for Anxiety-Related Conditions, Obsessive-Compulsive Disorder (OCD), & Post-Traumatic Stress Disorder (PTSD)

A) Breathing Exercise

(May be especially useful for panic; agoraphobia; generalized anxiety; phobias; social phobia/anxiety; post-traumatic & acute stress).

Shortness of breath is a common feeling that many people get when anxious. When one feels out of breath the natural tendency is to breathe in more or faster. This can lead to hyperventilation which can make anxiety worse.

An effective way to manage abnormal breathing when anxious is to do the following:

- Breathe in slowly to the count of three.

- Breathe using your <u>abdomen</u> instead of the chest.

- When you get to three, slowly breathe out to the count of three seconds.

- Pause for three seconds then breath in again for 3 seconds.

- Continue this exercise for five minutes.

- Practice twice a day.

B) Muscle relaxation exercise

(May be especially useful for panic; agoraphobia; generalized anxiety; social anxiety; post-traumatic & acute stress).

For each of the muscle groups in your body, tense the muscles for 5–10 seconds, then relax for 10 seconds. Only tense your muscles moderately (not to the point of inducing pain). Don't force the release of the muscle tension - simply let go of the tension in your muscles and allow them to become relaxed. Relax your muscles in the following order:

Hands — clench one fist tightly, then relax. Do the same with the other hand.

Lower arms — bend your hand down at the wrist, as though you were trying to touch the underside of your arm, then relax.

Upper arms — bend your elbows and tense your arms. Feel the tension in your upper arm, then relax.

Shoulders — lift your shoulders up as if trying to touch your ears with them, then relax.

Neck — stretch your neck gently to the left, then forward, then to the right, then to the back in a slow rolling motion, then relax.

Forehead and scalp — raise your eyebrows, then relax.

Eyes — look about, rotating your eyes, then relax.

Jaw — clench your teeth (just to tighten the muscles), then relax.

Tongue — press your tongue against the roof of your mouth, then relax.

Chest — breathe in deeply to inflate your lungs, then breath out and relax.

Stomach — suck your tummy in to tighten the muscle, then relax.

Upper back — pull your shoulders forward with your arms at your side, then relax.

Lower back — while sitting, lean your head and upper back forward, rolling your back into a smooth arc thus tensing the lower back, then relax.

Buttocks — tighten your buttocks, then relax.

Thighs — while sitting, push your feet firmly into the floor, then relax.

Calves — lift your toes off the ground towards your shins, then relax.

Feet — gently curl your toes down so that they are pressing into the floor, then relax.

Enjoy the feeling of relaxation: Take some slow breaths while you sit still for a few minutes, enjoying the feeling of relaxation.

Practice once or twice a day. During the day, try relaxing specific muscles whenever you notice that they are tense.

III: Conditions & Issues: Anxiety-Related Conditions, OCD, & PTSD

C) Problem-solving exercise

(May be especially useful for generalized anxiety & social anxiety).

Choose one or two problems that are particularly bothersome and make a decision to try to resolve them as best as possible.

1. On a sheet of paper, list the specific problems.

2. List five or six possible solutions to the problem. Write down any ideas that occur to you, not merely the 'good' ideas.

3. Evaluate the positive and negative points of each idea.

4. Choose the solution that best fits your needs.

5. Plan exactly the steps you will take to put the solution into action.

6. Review your efforts after attempting to carry out the plan. Praise all efforts. If unsuccessful, start again.

D) Managing negative, distorted thinking

(May be especially useful for generalized anxiety; social anxiety; & obsessive -compulsive disorder).

Significant anxiety can influence thoughts and emotions and progress to negative, pessimistic feelings and even irrational, distorted thoughts.

Management of negative distorted thoughts involves:

- Identifying the negative, distorted thoughts

- Substituting these thoughts with more realistic ideas (create a list of alternative thoughts that are realistic, positive and counter each negative thought listed). This is an important skill that can help reduce anxiety symptoms.

E) Graded exposure (Gradual exposure to feared objects or situations). *The relevance of the examples listed will vary among different cultures and societies.*

This may be particularly useful for phobias. It incorporates the breathing and relaxation exercises as well. The key strategy for overcoming fears of this kind involves creating a plan or hierarchy of steps. The individual is gradually exposed to the fearful object or situation, in small steps, so that eventually less anxiety is experienced when the object or situation is present. For example, a woman refuses to go on a public bus fearing that it will have an accident. However, she must use a bus to get to work and run important errands such as going to the market.

First – teach the breathing and relaxation exercises to the individual since these techniques will be important in reducing the anxiety felt during moments when an aspect of the frightening object or situation is present.

Second – clearly outline with the individual the steps of the exposure process:

- Start with a picture of the frightening object (bus).

- Look at pictures of a bus or take a trip to a bus stop without actually getting on the bus.

- Take a very brief bus ride (1 or 2 stops).

- Increase the amount of time on the bus.

During each step, the individual should be expressing his/her feelings, using breathing and relaxation to control anxiety occurring in the moment.

In separate sessions, use the exercise in "Managing Negative, Distorted Thinking" to correct thought distortions, misconceptions or fears about the object or situation.

Medication Therapy for Anxiety-Related Conditions, OCD, & PTSD

See "Medication Guide" section of the manual.

Somatic Symptom Disorder & Psychological Factors Affecting Other Medical Conditions

Somatic Symptom Disorder

Signs/characteristics

Given the connection between the mind (brain) and body, it is possible for individuals to express emotional distress as physical (somatic) symptoms. A somatic symptom disorder should be considered if one is excessively and persistently preoccupied with physical symptoms such that daily life and function are adversely affected.

Individuals with somatic symptom disorder may present with excessive thoughts, feelings, and behaviors associated with somatic symptoms. Constant anxiety about symptoms or health in general may be present, the seriousness of symptoms may be exaggerated and persistently emphasized, and excessive time and energy are spent focused on the symptoms. One somatic symptom (particularly pain) or more may be experienced and symptoms may or may not be associated with another medical condition. In severe cases, individuals may repeatedly visit health services, have a tendency to request only symptom relief, and have little ability to accept that no physical illness is present when diagnostic testing is unremarkable.

US studies have indicated that the prevalence of somatic symptom disorder is 5%-7% in the general adult population and females tend to report more somatic symptoms than do males. In addition, somatic symptom disorder is related to high rates of co-morbid conditions including anxiety, depression, and medical disorders.

III: Conditions & Issues: Somatic Symptom Disorder & Psychological Factors Affecting Other Medical Conditions

Counseling Interventions For Somatic Symptom Disorder

General considerations:

- Acknowledge that the individual's complaints are real but avoid recommending unnecessary or new medications for each new symptom if examinations and diagnostic tests are unremarkable.

- Ask the individual's opinion about potential causes of symptoms.

- Support the concept of wellness rather than a focus on symptoms and illness.

- Discuss emotional stress that may have accompanied symptoms originally. Explain that stress may be related to the physical symptoms experienced. A brief respite may be helpful for individuals complaining in relation to recent stress. If indicated, offer relaxation methods that can decrease tension.

- For individuals with chronic complaints schedule regular, time-limited appointments with the same clinician if possible.

Exercise

For individuals who have some insight about the connection between their emotions and physical complaints the following technique may be useful.

1. Have the individual list his/her physical complaints, severity of the complaints, activities involved in as physical problems are experienced, and the emotions that are occurring as the physical problems are experienced:

Physical problem	Severity of problem (scale of 1-10; 10=very severe)	Activities	Emotions
1. headache

2.

3. | 8 | Going to the market | irritable |

2. Explore with the individual, the possible connection between the physical complaint and emotions experienced.

3. Discuss possible ways to adjust the activities so that emotional distress is reduced (i.e. changing the day or time of day to a time when there are no other chores to do; reducing the amount done at one time in order to have more free time; using the help of others; incorporating a pleasurable activity into a trip to the market; praising and rewarding oneself for the efforts).

III: Conditions & Issues: Somatic Symptom Disorder & Psychological Factors Affecting Other Medical Conditions

Medication Therapy For Somatic Symptom Disorder

Medication Therapy for Somatic Symptom Disorder

1. Treatment of underlying/co-existing medical conditions is important.

2. Antidepressant and/or anti-anxiety medications for underlying/co-existing depression and/or anxiety is recommended.

See the "Medication Guide " section of the manual for medication therapy for depression and anxiety conditions.

Psychological Factors Affecting Other Medical Conditions

Signs/Characteristics

Psychological factors affecting other medical conditions involve the presence of one or more psychological or behavioral factors that negatively affect a medical condition by precipitating, exacerbating or increasing the severity and/or extent of illness (e.g. increased asthma symptoms after experiencing stress). Psychological/behavioral factors may include depression, anxiety, stressful life events, and maladaptive personality traits, coping style, and relationship style.

Counseling Interventions & Medication Therapy

Treatment involves stabilization of any medical symptoms present, use of anti-anxiety and antidepressant medication for co-existing anxiety disorders or depression, counseling, and psychotherapy.

Counseling interventions

See the previous section (Somatic Symptom Disorder) for a useful exercise.

Medication therapy

See the "Medication Guide " section of the manual for medication therapy for depression and anxiety conditions.

SUBSTANCE USE DISORDERS

Signs/Characteristics

A) Definitions regarding psychoactive substances (i.e. substances that activate the brain and cause effects on thoughts, emotions, and behaviors).

1. Intoxication – maladaptive behavior associated with recent drug ingestion.

2. Withdrawal – adverse physical & psychological symptoms that occur following cessation of the drug.

3. Tolerance – the need for more substance to attain the same level of effect.

4. Abuse or Misuse – a maladaptive pattern of use leading to repetitive problems and negative consequences (i.e. use in dangerous situations such as driving; use leading to legal, social and occupational problems).

5. Dependence (addiction) — continued desire for and use of a psychoactive substance to satisfy pleasurable urges and/or to alleviate the effects of withdrawal. Dependence may be psychological or physical in nature.

Psychological dependence:

- Persistent substance use, despite evidence of its harmful consequences.

- Difficulties in controlling the use of the substance.

- Neglect of interests and an increased amount of time taken to obtain the substance or recover from its effects.

- Evidence of tolerance such that higher doses are required to achieve the same effect.

- Compulsion or craving: a strong desire to take the substance.

- Anxiety or mood disturbance occurs if drug is not taken.

Physical dependence:

- Physical symptoms occur if drug is not taken (e.g. headache; gastrointestinal distress; changes in blood pressure, heart rate; sweating; tremors; muscular pain).

B) Effects of Selected Psychoactive Substances

Alcohol

Worldwide, alcohol consumption and problems related to alcohol vary widely, but , in most countries, the burden of disease and death remains significant. Alcohol consumption is the world's third largest risk factor for disease and disability behind high blood pressure (first) and smoking (second). In middle-income countries, it is the greatest risk. The world's highest alcohol consumption levels are found in developed countries.

Intoxication Symptoms: Slurred speech; unstable walking; mood change; aggression; anxiety; psychosis; sleep disturbance; and delirium.

Withdrawal Symptoms (occurring several hours to a few days after cessation of use that has been heavy and prolonged): Nausea; headache; nystagmus (rapid horizontal movement of eyeballs); unstable blood pressure or heart rate; psychosis; anxiety; mood disturbance; sleep disturbance; delirium; and seizure.

Cannabis

Worldwide, cannabis (with a global annual prevalence ranging from 2.6 to 5.0 per cent) remains the most widely used illicit drug according to the United Nations Office on Drugs and Crime (UNODC) 2012 report.

Intoxication Symptoms: Elevated or depressed mood; anxiety; inappropriate laughing; paranoia; hallucinations; red eyes; increased appetite; dry mouth; increased heart rate.

Studies have indicated an association between high doses of cannabis and delirium, panic, ongoing psychosis may occur. In addition, Longterm use has been linked to anxiety, depression, and loss of motivation.

Withdrawal Symptoms (occurring 1 week after cessation of prolonged, heavy use, i.e. a few months of daily or near daily use): Depressed or irritable mood; anxiety; restlessness; sleep disturbance; poor appetite; and weight loss.

C) Interventions for Substance Use Disorders

• Refer to medical evaluation, diagnosis, & medical stabilization as indicated.

• Assess for underlying psychiatric conditions (e.g. depression, anxiety).

• Refer to drug counseling program if available or psychological services for treatment.

Additional Counseling Interventions For Substance Use Disorders

1. Anxiety and depression may underlie substance abuse. Also, some individuals with bipolar disorder or a psychotic disorder may use alcohol or drugs to self-medicate or deal with symptoms. It is therefore important to evaluate for these psychiatric conditions and provide or refer to the appropriate treatments. For some individuals, drug and alcohol use is decreased if underlying anxiety, mood disturbance, or other distress is relieved.

2. Teach breathing and relaxation techniques as a means for controlling anxiety (see chapter on "Anxiety Disorders" for technique instructions).

3. Encourage individuals to identify people who can be contacted for support when cravings or distress occurs. Another who is also recovering from addiction and is sober can be a good ally.

NEUROCOGNITIVE DISORDERS:

DELIRIUM & DEMENTIA

The term "neurocognitive disorder" refers to a significant decline from a previous level of function in one or more of cognitive realms including awareness (orientation, consciousness), complex attention (sustained, selective, and divided attentions); executive function (planning, decision making, mental flexibility); learning and memory; language; perceptual-motor (visual perception and construction, integration of visual perception with movement); and social cognition (recognition of emotions, ability to consider other's mental state). Types of neurocognitive disorders include: 1) delirium and 2) major & mild neurocognitive disorders (dementia).

1) Delirium

Delirium is a disturbance particularly in the ability to focus, sustain, or shift attention. Other characteristics of delirium may include additional deficits in cognition (e.g. memory, perception), rapid onset, a fluctuating course, reversiblility, agitation, irritability, and psychosis (i.e. distortion of reality). Causes of delirium may include brain disease, systemic disease (e.g. heart disease), drugs, medications, and other toxins.

Neuropsychiatric symptoms of delirium may be identified through a thorough mental status examination. The underlying cause of disease may be identified, if resources are available, through a complete battery of laboratory and diagnostic tests [e.g. blood chemistries, complete blood count, chest x-ray, urinalysis & toxicology, electrocardiogram (EKG), computerized tomography (CT) scan, or magnetic resonance imaging of the brain].

2) Major/Mild Neurocognitive Disorder (Dementia)

Major neurocognitive disorder (dementia) may be difficult at times to differentiate from delirium, as there are a number of shared characteristics, particularly cognitive deficits (e.g. memory deficit). In general, a pervasive cognitive and intellectual decline with a lack of impaired awareness or consciousness is what distinguishes dementia from delirium. Other characteristics of the disorder may include slow onset; an ongoing, continuous course; irreversibility; agitation; irritability; depression; psychosis; and a gradual, permanent decline in function.

"Mild" neurocognitive disorder differs from the major disorder in the degree of disturbance present. Cognitive deficits are modest and do not interfere to a level where independent function is significantly impaired.

Conditions causing neurocognitive disorder include Alzheimer's disease, frontotemporal lobar degeneration, lewy body disease, vascular disease, brain trauma, brain tumors, infections (e.g. HIV), alcoholism, drug abuse, medications, other toxins, and poor oxygen supply.

A thorough mental status exam with particular attention to the evaluation of cognitive function will elucidate symptoms of major and mild neurocognitive disorder. Laboratory and diagnostic tests can identify underlying causes of disease.

INTERVENTIONS

Patients identified as having symptoms of delirium or dementia should be referred to the hospital for further evaluation, diagnosis, and treatment.

A) Delirium

· Adjust sensory stimulation as indicated (i.e. decrease stimulation if the person is agitated; increase if the person is sensory deprived).

· Place the person in an area that is safe and secure (no dangerous objects or hazards nearby) and where he/she can be observed easily.

B) Major/Mild Neurocognitive Disorders (Dementia)

· Arrange the environment so that there are clear cues for orientation to date, time, place.

· Incorporate proper nutrition, exercise, & mentally stimulating activity.

· Provide support for the family (e.g. education, group therapy).

Aids to enhance function:

Memory aids: Calendars; organizers; outline routines for daily activities; checklists; pill boxes; and timers.

Physical aids: Canes; wrist weights

Physical and mental stimulatory aids: Exercise such as walking, stretching, ball throwing; identify/encourage previous hobbies; card/board games; puzzles; encourage storytelling, singing; Encourage time with others who will stimulate (talkative friends).

Medications

Benzodiazepines and antipsychotics are used with caution to treat severe agitation associated with delirium. Antidepressants may be indicated for depressive symptoms associated with dementia. Elderly individuals with dementia-related psychosis treated with atypical antipsychotic medications are at an increased risk of death (due to infectious or cardiovascular conditions). HIV dementia may be treated and potentially reversed with antiretroviral therapy.

EPILEPSY

Epilepsy is a chronic disorder of the brain affecting approximately 50 million people in the world, with nearly 80% of the people with epilepsy found in developing countries. The condition is characterized by recurrent seizures (i.e. brief episodes of involuntary shaking) which may involve a part of the body (partial) or the entire body (generalized). Seizures are due to excessive electrical discharges within a network of brain cells and may be accompanied by loss of consciousness and control of bowel or bladder function.

Signs/characteristics of Epilepsy

The cause of epilepsy in 70% of cases is unknown. Other causes may include infection, brain injury, drugs/alcohol, vascular disease, or a nutrient imbalance. These conditions may cause "seizures" or destabilization and abnormal stimulation of nervous system cells. Seizures may be characterized as either partial (localized) or generalized (global):

1) Partial (focal) seizure – originates in a localized area and remains localized.

a) simple - consciousness is not affected (e.g. motor).

b) complex - some localized or specific areas of the brain may have more complex associations and function than other areas. Seizure activity within these circuits may result in "complex-localized" seizures.

81

Complex-localized seizures may be characterized by an "aura" or a set of abnormal sensory signals such as light flashes, smells and noises that precede the onset of a seizure. Consciousness may also be impaired with this type of seizure.

c) secondarily generalized – seizure spreads locally to generally.

2) Generalized seizure– originates centrally and continues generally (i.e. globally).

a) absence/petit mal (typical symptoms may include staring; stop mid-sentence then continue). May be typical or atypical in presentation.

b) tonic-clonic/grand mal (aura; all 4 limbs involved; unconscious; incontinence; post-ictal confusion, headache, or excessive sleep).

c) other generalized seizures include myoclonic (involuntary twitching of a muscle or group of muscles); clonic (involuntary rhythmic jerking); and atonic ("drop attack" or lapse of muscle tone).

Psychiatric Manifestations

Change in personality is common while psychosis and violence have been found to occur less frequently than previously perceived. Temporal lobe epilepsy has been associated with instability in mood.

Counseling Interventions For Epilepsy

1. Educate the family/caretakers. Review with them the signs and symptoms of epilepsy. Provide guidance on what to do if one has a seizure. Emphasize the importance of medication compliance. Explain to parents that epilepsy has been associated with behavioral change and conduct disturbance in children and provide them with guidance on how to set limits and reinforce constructive behaviors.

2. Help the individual identify situations that cause stress or anxiety as these can be triggers for a relapse of illness. Help the individual limit involvement in these situations or (if situation is unavoidable) help the individual think in advance about what will occur and how he/she will respond. Breathing and relaxation exercises can be incorporated to help reduce anxiety felt in these situations (see chapter on Anxiety-Related Conditions for breathing and relaxation exercises).

3. Emphasize keeping track of appointments. Missed appointments can lead to the individual's running out of medication. Missing doses of medicine can put him/her at risk for a return of symptoms and a relapse of illness.

4. Medication Compliance. The individual should discuss with the doctor medication options and regimens that will make taking pills easy (use pill organizer boxes; is once a day dosing possible?).

Medication Therapy

See "Medication Guide" section of the guide.

SLEEP DISTURBANCE

Signs/characteristics

A disturbance in sleep can occur as a part of or separately from a psychiatric condition. Studies from western cultures have indicated that insomnia (decreased ability to sleep) is common and can have many causes (e.g. as a primary condition or due to a secondary cause such as medical illness, psychiatric conditions, medications, or drugs and alcohol). Sleep disturbance is one of the commonest responses to stress.

Counseling Interventions For Sleep Disturbance

Sleep hygiene (measures to create a regular sleep pattern)

1) Set a regular bedtime and make efforts to adhere to it even if not tired.

2) Make efforts to arise at the same time each morning.

3) Avoid napping during the day.

4) Exercise during the day. Practice relaxation exercises in the evening (e.g. meditation, yoga).

5) Ensure a comfortable sleep space.

6) Limit activating substances (e.g. caffeine, alcohol, nicotine); none in the second half of the day is recommended.

7) Address any underlying medical or psychiatric disturbance.

Medication Therapy

See " Medication Guide" section of manual.

LOSS & BEREAVEMENT

Signs/Characteristics

Grief is the name for the feelings accompanying the loss of any loved person, place, or object. This can include one's home, one's health (e.g. being diagnosed with a long term illness or having a limb amputation) and one's country or culture (e.g. being a refugee).

Loss and the process of grieving (bereavement) is complex and will vary from one individual to the next. Emotional responses to loss, death and dying have been described by Kubler-Ross and include:

a) Denial – There is an inability to accept that the loss has occurred. This may be accompanied by a feeling of shock, surprise and numbness. One cannot believe that such a thing could happen to him/her.

b) Anger – anger and hostility may be experienced. Blaming others or oneself for not preventing the loss is a common theme.

c) Bargaining – belief that if one acts or thinks differently the loss can be retrieved (or in the case of dying, the loss can be avoided). One may feel severe guilt ("Maybe this would not have happened if I had been more attentive…").

d) Depression or emotional breakdown – the reality of the loss sets in. There can be feelings of unbearable loneliness, sadness, loss of motivation and interest; the person may withdraw from contact with others. Anxiety, panic, and thought disorganization can occur. Emotional distress may also be expressed as agitation, fatigue, impaired sleep, and impaired appetite.

87

e) Acceptance – one is able ultimately to place the loss in perspective and move on to new activities and relationships.

Initially, it was believed that these reactions occurred in a linear, stage-like fashion, however, responses do not have to follow an established order. The feeling may occur in rapid succession or in combination (e.g. depression and anger). In addition, caregivers to dying individuals may also experience these reactions.

A variety of factors may influence a person's ability to manage loss. These factors may include:

1. Age/emotional maturity.

2. Personality traits - capacity for resiliency, independence, disappointment, patience.

3. Belief systems - What does this loss represent? How does one view death – as a part of the life cycle or as a horrible event to be avoided? One may believe that the spirit of a deceased loved one can live on through the memories maintained by his/her survivors.

4. Psychological defense mechanisms - e.g. sublimating or neutralizing loss through humor or humanitarian actions.

5. Personal expectations.

6. Support system - family, friends, healthcare workers.

Counseling Interventions

Individuals will vary in the way and degree to which they grieve. People with prolonged distress or distress affecting their function should be evaluated for major depression and other psychological conditions.

The following general points may be useful in helping people through the grieving process:

1. Ensure that normal culturally appropriate mourning processes have been able to take place.

2. Provide reassurance that the grieving process is normal despite the painful feelings it causes. Do not force talking. People choose their own times and situations to share feelings – but make it clear that you can listen if they wish to share their painful experiences and feelings.

3. Encourage finding simple ways to enjoy positive memories of the past (e.g. through photographs and stories).

4. Provide reassurance that unbearable, painful feelings can decrease over time.

5. Recommend adequate rest and exercise.

6. Help the individual understand that it is not unusual for people to experience dreams, nightmares, visions or desire to talk to the dead.

7. Recommend avoiding making large, complex decisions.

8. Help the individual be aware that there may be events or circumstances when painful feelings about the loss are triggered (e.g. birthdays, anniversaries, other deaths, etc…). Being prepared for this will diminish the impact.

9. Help one understand that loss involves change and that new activities or relationships may be a part of the change.

III: Conditions & Issues: Loss & Bereavement

Loss & Bereavement in Children

A) General

Children at different stages of development have different reactions to loss. Some individuals may develop an understanding sooner or later than their peers, however, in general, children begin to develop an understanding of the finality of death around the age of five. Studies (western) indicate that children who suffer an early bereavement have a higher incidence of psychiatric disorders in later childhood. In addition, adults who are bereaved of a parent in childhood are more vulnerable to psychiatric disorders than the general population. When additional losses are experienced, they may be more prone to depression and anxiety than the general population.

B) Children Under Age 5

Under five, children do not understand the irreversibility of death. Children under five generally demonstrate unrealistic or "magical" thinking that results in misconceptions about causes and effects. They also have an egocentric or self-centered view of the world leading to a feeling of responsibility for a death (e.g. "Mommy won't come back because I was naughty..."). Reactions are similar to those following any separation where the longer the absence, the greater the distress. A child may appear detached as though he or she does not care.

C) Children Age 5 – 10years

After the age of five, children can understand that death is irreversible, however, they still may not regard it as something that can affect them. They may continue to have some magical, concrete, and egocentric thinking. Children at this age have a concept of good and bad, become curious about cause and effect, and are able to articulate concern for others. Children may express the desire to stay connected to the dead parent.

D) Age 10 - Adolescence

During this stage, children begin to develop an understanding of abstract concepts regarding death (e.g. death is universal and inevitable and can affect them personally). They also become aware of inconsistencies and can experience the conflict between concepts such as justice versus injustice and the desire for independence versus the need for closeness. Death can feel confusing and conflictual - individuals at this age may express feelings of indifference, detachment, identification, or nostalgia. Additional common immediate reactions to death for children in this age range are listed in the box below.

Common Immediate Reactions to Death/Loss (children age 10-adolescence)

Shock & disbelief	Guilt, self-reproach and shame
Dismay and protest	Physical complaints
Apathy and feeling stunned	School problems
Continuation of usual activities	Regressive behavior
Anxiety	Social isolation
Vivid memories	Fantasies
Sleep problems	Personality changes
Sadness and longing	Pessimism about the future
Anger and acting out behavior	Rapid maturing

E) Guidelines for Managing Loss & Bereavement in Children

When a child has experienced a loss, it is best not to hide the truth. Children need clear, honest, consistent explanations appropriate to their level of development. They need to accept the reality of the loss not to be protected from it. Magical thinking should be explored and corrected. What is imagined may be worse than reality and children may be blaming themselves for events beyond their control. Encourage a supportive environment where open communication is possible, difficult questions are answered, and distressing feelings are tolerated. Allow children to express grief in a manner they find appropriate, to express to the people they most trust and feel comfortable, and to express at a time of their choosing.

If a child has lost a parent or significant caretakers, the child will need to be provided consistent, enduring, appropriate care. The more continuity with the child's previous life, the better. Children may wish to avoid traumatic reminders, especially in the beginning, but complete removal from a familiar environment may cause more pain and problems in the long term. They should be reunited with caring extended family if available.

III: Conditions & Issues: Loss & Bereavement

Loss & Bereavement in Disasters/Catastrophic Emergencies

A disaster or catastrophic emergency may be defined as a significant nature-related (e.g. earthquakes, tsunami, hurricanes, floods, etc) or human-related event (e.g. armed conflict) that directly threatens life or compromises the basic needs required to sustain life (i.e. food, shelter, water & sanitation, security, disease control, or access to health care). Losses and grief under these circumstances can be devastating and overwhelming. There may be formal supportive efforts provided by various humanitarian organizations or less formal support by individuals and other neighboring communities.

For organizations lending aid, the Inter-agency Standing Committee (IASC) Task Force on Mental Health and Psychosocial Support has developed guidelines for primary (acute phase) and secondary/comprehensive (reconsolidation phase) social and psychological interventions that may be useful in helping individuals and communities recover constructively (see the chapter, "An Approach to Care: Crisis Situations—Disaster/Emergency Settings").

MATERNAL MENTAL HEALTH

Maternal mental health disorders are a public health challenge posing a significant personal, social, and economic burden on women, their babies, their families, and society. Studies indicate that depression and anxiety are about two times as prevalent worldwide in women than in men and tend to occur at their highest rates during childbearing years (i.e. puberty to menopause). The incidence of depression and anxiety is highest in the year following delivery compared to during pregnancy or at a time of no pregnancy. In developed countries, suicide is one of the most common causes of maternal death during the year after delivery. While psychosis post-partum is uncommon, in developing countries, rates may be higher (due to infection as a contributing factor).

Risk Factors for Developing Mental Health Disorders (during pregnancy and in the first year following delivery)

1. poverty
2. extreme stress
3. exposure to domestic, gender-based, or sexual violence
4. limited social support network
5. natural disasters or emergency & conflict situations migration

Pregnancy & Mental Health

While the majority of women cope well with the changes associated with pregnancy and motherhood, some experience distress that can potentially affect the health of both mother and child. Major depression and some anxiety disorders are common in the general population and may also be seen in pregnant women.

Other issues that may occur as a result of maternal mental disorders during pregnancy include poor sleep, poor eating and inadequate weight gain, increase in stress hormone potentially (causing high blood pressure, pre-eclampsia, & early/ complicated delivery for the mother and impaired growth for the developing baby), poor motivation to seek prenatal, perinatal, and postnatal care, and alcohol and other substance abuse (e.g. cigarettes, illicit drug).

Although conditions such as depression and anxiety may be treated with medication, drugs are used with significant caution during pregnancy. There have been studies with some antidepressant agents that indicate efficacy but these studies are very limited and still advise caution due to the potential risk to the fetus.

Helping the mother make lifestyle adjustments and utilize the support of family, friends, and educational resources is highly emphasized. Prevention is important - a healthcare provider who is able to identify depressive or anxiety symptoms early and provide support can reduce a mother's potential for developing a depressive or anxiety disorder.

Post - Partum Conditions

The mother may experience distress following the delivery of the child. Conditions after birth may include post-partum sadness (also known as post-partum "blues"), post-partum depression, or post-partum psychosis. Specific symptoms and management of these conditions are outlined in the table on the following page.

Maternal mental disorders may have a significant effect not only on the mother but also on the infant and other family members. For example, depression and anxiety in the mother may lead to poor mother-infant attachment, affecting the child's social, emotional, and cognitive development. In addition, marital problems including disruption of marriage and abuse by the partner may occur as a result of mental illness in a mother after childbirth.

III: Conditions & Issues: Maternal Mental Health

Post Partum Conditions

Condition	Symptoms	Management
Post-partum Sadness or "Blues"	Common; Mildly depressed mood, irritability, anxiety, insomnia, tearfulness (often 1-10 days after delivery)	Symptoms remit spontaneously but educate mother and family that this occurrence is common; however, symptoms persisting beyond 2 weeks should be evaluated (for the possibility of a depressive disorder).
Post-partum Depression	Sadness; anger; insomnia; fatigue; impaired sleep; impaired appetite; decreased sexual interest; crying spells without obvious cause; worthlessness; hopelessness; poor memory and concentration.	Creating a supportive environment for the mother; encouraging self-care. Counseling and education about symptoms; monitor for suicidal thoughts; antidepressant medication if symptoms are severe and persistent (take caution with mothers who are breast-feeding). See section on "Mood Disorders - Depression" for treatment.
Post-partum Psychosis	Uncommon; disorganized thought; delusions that the child may be defective or dying, or that he or she is not her real child. She may also have ideas of killing her child to protect him against illogical threats.	Education about symptoms; monitor for homicidal thoughts; anti-psychotic medication only for severe, persistent psychotic symptoms (take caution with mothers who are breast-feeding). See section on "Psychotic Disorders" for treatment.

MENTAL HEALTH ISSUES IN CHILDREN

1.   Neurodevelopmental Disorders

The neurodevelopmental disorders are conditions that tend to occur early in the developmental period and may include impairments in intelligence, executive function, learning, and social skills. Personal, social, academic, and occupational functioning may be limited with some disorders manifesting with deficits and delays in reaching normal developmental milestones. Symptoms often occur prior to a child's entering grade school and often occur co-morbidly with other neurodevelopmental disorders.

The Diagnostic & Statistical Manual of Mental Disorders-Fifth Edition (DSM-V) classifies neurodevelopmental disorders into categories including intellectual disabilities, communication disorders, autism spectrum disorder (ASD), attention-deficit/ hyperactivity disorder (ADHD), specific learning disorder, motor disorders, and other neurodevelopmental disorders. In this chapter, specific conditions that are emphasized include intellectual developmental disorder, autism spectrum disorder, ADHD, and Tourette's disorder (motor disorder).

A) Intellectual Disability (intellectual developmental disorder)

Intellectual disability, or intellectual developmental disorder, is a condition of disabled mental abilities, such as reasoning, problem solving, planning, abstract thinking, judgment, academic learning, and learning from experience. An individual's adaptive functioning in daily life may be impaired such that he or she is unable to become an independent and responsible member of society.

The global prevalence of intellectual disability is about two out of every hundred persons. Prenatal causes of intellectual disability include genetic syndromes, inborn errors of metabolism, brain malformations, maternal disease, and environmental influences. Perinatal and postnatal causes have included complications during labor and delivery, oxygen deprivation, traumatic brain injury, infections, demyelinating disorders, seizure disorders, severe and chronic social deprivation, and toxic metabolic syndromes and intoxications. A diagnosis of intellectual disability requires that an individual has impaired intellectual and adaptive functioning relative to the individual's age, gender, and socio-culturally matched peers. The onset of these deficits is during the developmental period before adulthood. Treatments for intellectual disability include early behavioral intervention, special education, specialized services, adaptive skill training, and transition planning.

B) Autism Spectrum Disorder

Autism spectrum disorder is a condition of impaired social communication and social interaction and the presence of restricted, repetitive patterns of behavior, interests or activities. Across US and non-US countries, the prevalence of autism spectrum disorder is approximately 1% of the population. Many factors may place a child at risk for autism spectrum disorder, such as advanced parental age, low birth weight, premature birth, or fetal exposure to valproic acid. Twin concordance studies have indicated heritability estimates ranging from 37% to 90% . Various genetic mutations have also been suggested as a contributing factor in some cases. A diagnosis of autism spectrum disorder is considered with the occurrence of continual deficits in reciprocal social communication and interaction and patterns of behavior, interests, or activities that are significantly restricted or repetitive. Symptoms begin during early childhood and hinder daily functioning. Effective treatments for autism spectrum disorder are early intervention services including applied behavioral analysis.

Dealing with intellectual disability and autism spectrum disorder: general points

Intellectual disability and autism spectrum disorder are chronic conditions. It is possible to help both the child and family make adaptations in their environment and interactions that will facilitate stable functioning. It is important to make a thorough evaluation of the child's psychiatric history (especially the developmental history) and perform a mental status examination. Be sure to ask about relatives who have had a similar condition.

Educate the family about the fact that the child has both limitations and potential. If available, seek evaluation by a specialist who can provide additional input on the specific diagnosis, degree of limitations, and the appropriate interventions. The important tasks will be accepting what the child cannot do and encouraging the development of skills the child possesses and can further develop.

Because comorbidity may occur with other neurodevelopmental, mental, and medical conditions (e.g. intellectual disability can be associated with conditions such as hyperactivity, depression, and epilepsy) inquire about these problems and provide or refer them to the appropriate treatment.

The family should provide structure by organizing a routine schedule for the child to follow that is appropriate to the child's level of function. This routine will help the child know what to expect and what to do – this can minimize anxiety and distress. The schedule should include a list of core activities of daily living that are appropriate to level of function so that basic self-care skills are fostered and maintained (e.g. washing; dressing; keeping the room tidy; food preparation, going to the market).

Include chores appropriate to the level of function so that a sense of responsibility is maintained. Whenever possible, have the child be actively involved in deciding work and pleasure activities. Be sure there is a good balance between indoor and outdoor activities. Also be sure to incorporate activities that involve social interaction.

Fostering "protective" factors can prevent the deterioration of a child's condition and help children to achieve their goals. Important protective factors include good physical health, healthy parent-child attachment, and a cohesive family unit within a supportive social network.

C) Attention Deficit/Hyperactivity Disorder (ADHD)

ADHD may be defined as a persistent pattern of inattention and/or hyperactivity-impulsivity that causes significant impairment in social or academic (occupational for adults) function (or marked distress) and is more frequent and severe than is typically observed in individuals at a comparable level of development.

ADHD occurs in approximately 5% of children and 2.5% of adults in most cultures, according to population surveys. Sources have indicated that low birth weight, premature delivery, smoking and alcohol use during pregnancy, exposure to environment toxicants, and brain injury are factors that have been variably correlated with ADHD, but are not known to be causal. ADHD heritability rates are rather high and specific genes have been correlated with the disorder.

Signs/Characteristics

Symptoms may exist as inattention singly or as hyperactivity/impulsivity, or a combination of inattention + hyperactivity/impulsivity. Symptoms of ADHD usually become apparent in primary school or other environments that are structured settings demanding task completion. In the school setting, teachers' observations are important. Teachers are in a position to compare patterns of compliance, on-task behavior, capacity for fundamental learning tasks (e.g. reading, spelling, arithmetic) and disruptiveness with other children pursuing similar tasks. A diagnosis of ADHD requires a continuous pattern of inattention and/or hyperactivity-impulsivity that negatively affects an individual's functioning or development.

105

Specific symptoms related to <u>inattention</u> may include:

- Poor attention to detail in work, school, and activities.

- Not attentive when spoken to.

- Easily distracted by external stimuli.

- Forgetfulness.

- Inconsistent follow through or execution of tasks and activities.

- Tendency to lose items associated with tasks or activities to be completed.

- Problem organizing activities or tasks.

- Tendency to dislike activities that require the capacity to be attentive.

- Impaired school performance and fundamental learning skills (e.g. reading, spelling, arithmetic) as a result of poor attention capacity

Specific symptoms related to <u>hyperactivity</u> and <u>impulsivity</u> include:

- Inability to sit quietly or be at rest when appropriate to do so.

- Excessive physical activity (e.g. climbing, running, jumping) when not appropriate.

- Speaking excessively.

- Tendency to interrupt or intrude on others' activities.

- Tendency to speak or act out of turn .

Reminder:

Not every child with problems at school or increased energy or activity level is considered to have ADHD. It is considered a problem ONLY if there is <u>continuing</u> interruption in school achievement or appropriate social interaction.

Management of ADHD

Avoid physical punishment as it aggravates the problem - rewarding the child for good behavior is more effective. Never give the child two tasks at the same time (i.e. give him or her one play activity or one toy at a time).

Educate the family that the child has a problem, needs help, and that patience is necessary. However, help the family also understand that they should not shy away from setting limits and should not be manipulated by the child. Teach the family interventions such as how to structure the child's day and organize his or her activities. Stimulant medications (e.g. methylphenidate) should be considered only if the problem persists and interferes with function and the child has shown no response to behavioral interventions.

Management – Structuring the Child's Day

Children with ADHD may need help in organizing, therefore:

- Schedule. Have the same routine every day, from wake-up time to bedtime. The schedule should include home-work time and playtime (including outdoor recreation and indoor activities). If a schedule change must be made, make it as far in advance as possible.

- Organize needed everyday items. Have a place for every-thing and keep everything in its place. This includes clothing, backpacks, and school supplies.

- Use homework and notebook organizers. Stress the im-portance of writing down assignments and bringing home needed books.

- Children with ADHD need consistent rules. Set consis-tent rules that they can understand and follow. If rules are followed, give a token of praise. Children with ADHD often receive, and expect criticism. Look for good behav-ior and praise it.

D) Tourette's Disorder

Tourette's disorder is a condition of multiple motor and vocal tics that occur for at least 1 year in variable frequencies. Tics are sudden, rapid, recurrent, nonrhythmic motor movements or vocalizations. The global prevalence of Tourette's disorder ranges from 1 to 30 per 1,000 persons according to studies. Research suggests Tourette's disorder is an inherited disorder, for which specific genes have been identified. Risk factors may include birth complications, older paternal age, lower birth weight, and maternal smoking or alcohol consumption during pregnancy.

A diagnosis of Tourette's disorder requires the presence of multiple motor tics and one or more vocal tics that occur for at least 1 year, and begin before age 18 years. Also, the tics cannot be due to substance use or another medical condition. Medication and behavioral therapy help to treat tics that cause physical injury or pain, or that interfere with daily functioning. However, some individuals have tics that do not interfere with their daily functioning and do not need treatment.

2. Emotional and Behavioral Problems

A) Depression and anxiety

Depression and some anxiety disorders are common in the adult population but occur with notable frequency in children as well. Depression and anxiety may coexist and, as with other conditions, may be expressed differently from one individual to the next. These conditions may be expressed in behavior or other nonverbal expressions, since children are at an early stage in their emotional maturity. A depressed child may appear sad, angry or agitated and may isolate from others. Children with anxiety, depression or a combination of both may also experience sleep problems or exhibit poor performance in school.

Management of depression or anxiety in children involves providing support for the child and education for the family. Antidepressant medications are not recommended for children (some medicines have been shown to increase distress and ideas of suicide) and many short-term anti-anxiety medicines have potential for addiction. Help the child and family identify the actions that may represent the distress and help them to identify the circumstances in which these actions occur. Even though a child's emotions are developing he or she can still be taught basic ways to verbalize distress. Using simple culturally appropriate picture charts showing different emotions and situations with which the child can identify, can be a way to begin discussions about feelings. Encourage the verbalization of distress. Verbalization can improve another's (family, schoolmates, teachers) ability to understand the child's problem and provide a more effective response. Help the child recognize and understand that negative feelings such as anger and disappointment are natural human emotions and that there are constructive ways to manage these emotions (i.e. help the child to identify and anticipate difficult situations and teach the child a variety of healthy responses to the situations).

It is equally important to help caretakers with distress obtain support, as children's emotions can often reflect the emotional climate within their environment. For example, a depressed parent may not have the energy or motivation to attend to the child's basic emotional needs. This can turn into psychological distress and emotional problems for the child.

B) Elimination Disorders

Enuresis (bed-wetting)

Enuresis may be defined as the inability of the child to control his bladder (after 5 years of age). The condition is not related to a secondary cause (such as a medical problem or ingestion of diuretic agents) but is psychological in nature. Enuresis may occur during sleep or while awake. Enuresis causes a lot of stress and shame for the child and can lead to more serious problem if not treated early. A thorough psychiatric history, mental status examination with emphasis on the developmental history, medical history, and social environment is important.

Management of Enuresis

A medical evaluation should be done to eliminate underlying medical causes for the problem. Be sure to assess for environmental conditions (e.g. if the wetting occurs during school time, is it due to dirty toilets, or unavailable toilets at school?). Also assess for other underlying psychological distress (e.g. the child who wets the bed may experience nightmares or night terrors and may be too afraid to go to the toilet).

Helpful Techniques

- Avoid bedtime fluid intake.

- The child should avoid an excess of foods or drinks that can stimulate urination (diuretics).

- The child should be taught to empty the bladder before going to sleep. Exercises to strengthen the bladder musculature may be used as well (e.g. start urination for 2-3 seconds, then stop the urination and hold for 5 seconds. Then resume and complete urination. Practicing this action each time the child must urinate can help to strengthen the muscles that control urine outflow).

- If the child is old enough, involve him/her in washing the bed sheets or clothes to decrease guilt and increase a sense of control and worth (sometimes the child has guilt believing that he/she causes inconvenience or distress for others).

- Another intervention that encourages self-esteem, self-control and self- worth is a calendar or chart that indicates progress in the child's decreased bed-wetting behavior. Instructions for creating the chart are outlined on the next page.

Monitoring Bed-wetting – the progress chart/calendar

- Make an attractive chart for the child that includes the days of the week (or use a calendar).

- Make the design simple since it is the child who will be actively filling in the chart.

- Have the child mark √ for the dry days and X for wet days (try to use the expressions "wet and dry" to minimize the stigma of the problem).

- To make it more fun, you can also have the child color the dry days with green and the wet days with red (or draw a sun for dry and clouds for wet etc…).

- At the end of each week ask the child to count dry and wet days and give him a reward for each improvement (e.g. if he had 5 wet days on the first week and 4 on second then offer a token of praise. If he maintains this improvement for 2 weeks continue to reward him; with additional improvement offer additional rewards).

- If after one month you are not getting benefits, reconsider underlying causes and another medical work-up.

Progress Chart for Monitoring Bedwetting

Mon	Tues	Wed	Thurs	Fri	Sat	Sun

C) Conduct Disorder

Conduct disorder may be defined as a persistent or repetitive pattern of behavior that involves aggression toward people or animals, destruction of property, deceitfulness or theft, and serious violations of well-established rules or social norms. Conduct disorder in children has been associated with infant temperament, lower-than-average intelligence, and instability in the family. In addition, violent behaviors have been correlated with physical or sexual abuse and alcoholism or drug use within the family.

An assessment not only of the child but also of the family and other environmental influences will elucidate information that will guide treatment. Education on how to identify and express emotions may be useful to the child and families. Alcohol and drug treatment should be recommended to those in need. Threats to a child's safety should be reported to the appropriate authorities.

ADOLESCENT PSYCHOSOCIAL ISSUES

Neuropsychiatric disorders are a leading cause of health-related burden for youth, accounting for 15–30% of the disability-adjusted life-years (DALYs) lost during the first three decades of life. With regard to the global perspective (particularly regarding low and middle-income countries), important psychosocial issues in adolescents have included substance abuse, violent behavior, and unsafe sexual behavior.

Substance Abuse

Risk factors associated with adolescent substance abuse include:

- Male gender

- Youth

- Genetics

- Mental health

- Poor personal/social skills

- Family dysfunction

- Dysfunctional peer group

- Limited educational or occupational opportunities

Peer pressure, excitement/enjoyment, self image, risk taking/ rebellion, curiosity, and experimentation are reasons cited by youth to use substances.

117

Factors that may be protective include a supportive family, individual motivation, high self esteem, and low motivation for impulsivity. In addition, having educational or occupational opportunities and an interest and capacity for socialization may reduce the risk for engaging in substance abuse.

Intervention:

- Evaluate mental and medical status

- Stabilize acute psychiatric and medical conditions

- Assess for underlying chronic psychiatric conditions; assess current social situation

- Provide information – regarding effects of drug

- Provide support – offer encouragement and referral to supportive services

Violence & Adolescents

From a global perspective, studies have indicated that violent death is not uncommon among adolescents and young adults. Among youth 10-29 years of age worldwide, each year approximately 250 000 homicides occur, constituting 41% of the annual total number of homicides globally. Social, political, and economic upheaval may be strong predictors of youth conflict (as opposed to poverty alone). In addition, adolescent girls (age 12-17) may be at particular risk for being sexually violated.

118

Risk Factors for Violence:

1) Individual Factors

- Gender

- Age

- Gang membership

- Psychiatric factors

- History of victimization

- Social dysfunction

- Drug use

2) Interpersonal Factors

- Exposure to violence

3) Community Factors

- Neighborhood deprivation

4) Societal Factors

- Culture of violence

- Social & economic inequality

Managing Adolescent Violence

Dealing with youth violence involves continued research that will help guide effective interventions. Development and government agencies will need to play a role in establishing policies which serve to change cultural and social norms that support violence. Raising awareness of the health consequences of youth violence and the importance of prevention is an important focus. Youth violence prevention policies and programs should be created. Specific preventive measures may include developing life skills in children and adolescents, decreasing the availability and harmful use of alcohol, and decreasing access to lethal means (e.g. guns, knives, pesticides).

Victims/Survivors of Violence

Youth are especially vulnerable regarding violence given their level of dependence, limited capacity to protect themselves, and limited power and participation in decision-making processes. Health care providers, relief workers and protection officers should devote special attention to their psychosocial needs.

Interventions for victims/survivors of violence:

- Protection

- Medical support as indicated

- Psychosocial support

- Monitoring by health facilities

- Education (i.e. individuals, families, communities)

Unsafe Sexual Behavior

Studies suggest evidence of high risk behavior among youth (e.g. being sexually active at a young age and irregular use of condoms). Factors that promote or perpetrate unsafe sexual behavior have included: personal factors; proximal environment; distal or broader social context; and interaction among factors.

1) Personal factors:

- Knowledge & beliefs

- Perception of low personal risk

- Self expectations

- Perceived costs & benefits

- Intentions

- Self-esteem

III: Conditions & Issues: Adolescent Psychosocial Issues

2) Proximal Environment:

Interpersonal Factors	Immediate Living Environment
• Negotiating condom use • Coercive, male-dominated sexual relationships • Peer pressure • Interactions with adult	• Lack of access to condoms • Low access to media • Lack of recreational facilities • Living on the street • Being in prison

3) Broader Social Context

   a) Culture

   b) Societal structure

     * urban vs rural conditions

     * poverty

4) Interaction among factors

III: Conditions & Issues: Adolescent Psychosocial Issues

Interventions:

- Psychosocial/psychiatric & medical assessments

- Provide factual information regarding safe sex practices

- Referral to supportive services

CRISIS SITUATIONS

1) AGITATION & AGGRESSIVE BEHAVIOR

Potential Causes

- Uncontrolled psychiatric condition such as mania, bipolar disorder, or psychosis.

- Untreated medical condition affecting the brain as an infection, tumor, or metabolic disease.

- Medication toxicity caused by an excessive amount or variety of medicines ingested.

- Alcohol or drug intoxication and withdrawal.

Intervention for Agitation/Aggression

- Alert and elicit the help of other healthcare staff or authorities.

- Take distance and help others remain a safe distance from the agitated person.

- Safety – if possible, try to remove from the environment items that are potentially hazardous to safety. Remain calm and confident.

- Listen, pay attention, do not argue.

- If possible (without subjecting yourself to harm) try to talk down or deescalate the individual by using a soft speech tone, expressing support and reassurance, and minimizing physical gestures.

2) SUICIDE

Risk Factors (western studies)

- Age (15-24yrs; elderly)
- Male gender
- Intense, prolonged suicidal thinking
- Past suicidal behavior

General questions to ask about suicide:

Do you feel very sad?

Do you feel that no one cares about you?

Do you feel you cannot go on?

Do you feel that life is not worth living?

Do you sometimes wish you were dead?

Have you thought of ending your life?

Are you having such thoughts now?

How often?

Have you actually made any plan?

Intervention for High risk Suicide (The person has a definite plan & the means to do it immediately).

- Stay with the person. Never leave the person alone.

- Gently talk to the person and remove the pills, knife, gun, insecticide, etc. (distance the means of suicide).

- Contact a mental health professional immediately, if available; Contact the local emergency services (or police) if mental health professionals are not available; Arrange for an ambulance and hospitalization.

- Contact the family or others significant to the individual and enlist their support.

- If a professional is not available for ongoing support, arrange future meetings at regular intervals and maintain ongoing contact.

3) DISASTER/EMERGENCY SETTINGS

A. General

Disasters or emergencies may be defined from different perspectives and have been characterized based on their potential for causing:

- Overwhelming physical environmental damage.

- Significant human morbidity or mortality.

- Impaired psychosocial function of individuals and communities.

- Impaired economic capacity of individuals or communities.

- Mobilization of revenue by organizations or government agencies to provide relief.

A disaster/emergency may be defined as a significant nature-related (e.g. earthquakes, tsunami, hurricanes, floods, etc) or human-related event (e.g. armed conflict)) that directly threatens life or compromises the basic needs required to sustain life (i.e. food, shelter, water & sanitation, security, disease control, or access to health care).

Disaster/emergency <u>relief</u> is defined in this text as the relief or assistance provided by various organizations or agencies in response to a nature-related or human-related emergency.

B. Phases of disaster/emergency relief & mental health interventions

A disaster or emergency relief effort may be described in terms of phases that include an acute **emergency phase** and **post-emergency or reconsolidation phase**. An affected population may experience varied degrees or fluctuate between phases depending on regional circumstances. The acute emergency phase has been defined as the period where crude mortality rate is increased due to circumstances or an environment in which basic needs (i.e. food, shelter, security, water/sanitation, disease control, and access to health care) are diminished.

During the emergency phase the focus is primarily on social interventions such as restoration of basic needs (i.e. food, shelter, security, water/sanitation, disease control, and access to health care). Psychological and psychiatric interventions during this phase are aimed at acute situations: the relief of acute distress through psychological first aid (see the next page); evaluation and treatment of severe conditions including suicidal intentions, psychosis, mania, severe depression, and epilepsy; and ensuring the availability of psychotropic medications for patients with pre-existing psychiatric conditions.

III: Conditions & Issues: Crisis Situations

Elements of Psychological First Aid (Sources: IASC Task Force on Mental Health & Psychosocial Support, 2007)

Elements Of Psychological First Aid

- Allowing survivors to discuss the events if they desire, without pressure; respect one's wish not to talk.

- Listening.

- Conveying compassion.

- Assessing and addressing basic needs (i.e. shelter, food, protection, health care, etc...).

- Discuss ways to manage or cope with stress (discourage destructive actions such as alcohol or substance abuse; encourage culturally appropriate constructive normal daily activities).

- Encouraging but not forcing company from significant others.

- If available, refer to local support mechanisms/mental health clinicians particularly if distress has been severe and sustained.

- Minimize the use of anti-anxiety medicines such as benzodiazepines which can be addictive (e.g. diazepam or alprazolam). If anxiety is severe and sustained (such that ability to function or manage self care is impaired) **short-term** use of an anti-anxiety medicine on an **as needed** basis can be used (i.e. start by giving a three day supply and instruct the individual to only use medicine in moments of overwhelming distress). Refer individuals with severe or sustained distress for further psychiatric evaluation and treatment if resources are available. Do not institute therapies or medications that require long-term or ongoing monitoring if no mechanism for monitoring (i.e. facilities or mental health staff trained to follow up) is established and available.

The post-emergency or reconsolidation phase has been defined as the period when basic needs have been restored to pre-emergency levels or to a standard within the population that represents a stable health condition. Emergency phase social, psychological, and psychiatric interventions are continued as needed during this phase. Post-emergency social interventions are focused on outreach and education while psychological and psychiatric evaluation and treatment services are further integrated into the existing primary health care structure.

GENDER-BASED VIOLENCE

IN INSECURE SETTINGS

Overview

In this discussion, an insecure setting is comparable to an emergency/ disaster relief (or humanitarian emergency) setting which may include communities uprooted or displaced by war, communities affected by natural disasters, or communities that have lost their integrity or structure due to other destabilizing circumstances. Gender-based violence (GBV) has been associated with insecure settings. Because of the serious nature and impact of GBV, the subject is addressed exclusively in this chapter.

The data on the prevalence and incidence of GBV in insecure settings have limitations due to under-reporting of incidents. Under-reporting occurs for many reasons including fear of retaliation and re-victimization, stigma, self blame, and mistrust of authorities. Data available on GBV have indicated, a female victim and male perpetrator are involved most frequently. While men and boys may also be vulnerable to sexual violence (particularly in situations of torture and detention) the majority of survivors/victims of sexual violence have been females.

Because there is a tendency for under-reporting, it is important that healthcare staff working in unstable environments have an awareness and willingness to take constructive action when violence is suspected. This chapter provides an outline of information on the nature, causes, effects, and active interventions associated with gender-based violence in insecure settings.

III: Conditions & Issues: Gender-Based Violence

Definitions & Causes of Gender-Based Violence (GBV)

Gender– based violence (GBV) has been defined broadly as any harmful act that is imposed against an individual's will, and that is based on socially ascribed (gender) differences between males and females. Specific types of GBV may vary across countries, regions, and cultures and may include: a) domestic violence; b) forced/early marriage; c) harmful traditional practices (e.g. female genital mutilation, honor killings, widow inheritance); d) trafficking; and e) sexual violence.

Regarding sexual violence, it may be described as an unwanted, destructive sexual advance that is executed (e.g. as a sexual action) or implied (e.g. as sexual verbal expression). Studies have indicated that power and control underlie the perpetration as opposed to an amorous attraction or desire. Forms of sexual violence seen in insecure settings have included: rape (most often cited); attempted assaults; verbal sexual threats and humiliating comments; molestation or repeated unwanted advances; domestic violence toward a spouse; and incest toward a family relative.

Reports have indicated that groups associated with GBV perpetration in insecure settings may include fellow refugees; other clan members; religious or ethnic groups; military personnel; relief workers; and family members. Regarding sexual violence, the survivor often knows the perpetrator.

134

Potential factors contributing to gender-based violence (GBV) in insecure settings

A) Displacement and the loss of community structures (due to social and armed conflict; natural disaster; or poverty and limited social and economic resources). Women and children may become separated from family and community supports, rendering them vulnerable to exploitation and abuse.

B) In conflict situations, women and children may be targeted particularly and GBV may be used as a tool for interrogation. Power and domination are employed with an intent to intimidate, humiliate, and control or hurt others. Abduction and sexual slavery occur in this setting.

C) Local populations may perceive refugees who receive special aid as privileged and therefore attack.

D) Male disrespect toward women leading to inequity in providing women food, shelter, security, and other necessities.

E) As a means for survival, women may be in the vulnerable position of bartering sex for food, shelter, and other necessities putting them at risk for abuse and violence.

Effects of GBV

The effects of GBV may manifest as medical, psychological, social, and economic problems:

A) *Medical*: sexually transmitted disease (e.g. syphilis, HIV); damage to the reproductive tract and susceptibility to chronic infections leading to pelvic inflammatory disease; unwanted pregnancy; unsafe abortion; and death from injuries.

B) *Psychological*: depression; terror; guilt; shame; loss of self-esteem; and suicide.

C) *Social*: rejection by a spouse, family, and community; loss of relationship with children.

D) *Economic*: loss of home, property, and security provided by family.

Active Interventions for GBV Incidents

In an insecure setting, efforts should be made, if possible, to identify and help coordinate local resources for protection, medical care, and psychosocial care.

1) Protection:

    A) Maintain confidentiality.

    B) Give individuals privacy, do not force them to express more than they desire, and reassure that they are in a safe setting while with you.

    C) Allow the individual to have family or friends be present if desired; if the incident has been recent, be aware that a medical evaluation may be required.

    D) Contact the police if the individual is amenable.

2) Medical Care – refer and provide an escort to medical care as indicated.

In cases of sexual assault/rape it is important to be aware of local and national laws (where they exist) and the procedures to collect forensic evidence as indicated. Procedures often indicate that the survivor should not wash, urinate, defecate, or change clothes before the medical exam in order to preserve important evidence.

A complete history of the incident and a physical examination should be conducted. As indicted, the history should include the nature of sexual contact, menstrual history, and mental state. The physical exam should note the condition of clothing, presence of foreign materials, evidence of physical trauma, and, as indicated, involve the collection of materials such as hair particles, fingernail scrapings, sperm, saliva, and blood samples.

Tests and treatments as indicated (e.g. tests for pregnancy, HIV, and syphilis; appropriate treatments for medical issues) should be provided. In addition, comprehensive counseling and follow-up medical care should be offered.

3) Psychosocial care

Reactions to GBV

Common reactions to GBV include fear, guilt, shame and anger. Survivors may adopt strong defense mechanisms that include forgetting, denial and deep repression of the events. Reactions vary from minor depression, grief, anxiety, phobia, and somatic problems to serious and chronic mental conditions. Extreme reactions to sexual violence may result in suicide or, in the case of pregnancy, physical abandonment or elimination of the child.

Supportive Counseling

Objectives of supportive counseling include helping survivors to understand what they have experienced, to express and place in perspective negative emotions, and to access support networks and services. Specific counseling points may include:

- Asking questions in a non-judgmental, non-intrusive, relevant manner; also, be aware that details and the sequence of information may change as the emotional state changes.

- If self-blame emerges, reassure the survivor that the perpetrator is to blame.

- Assess needs or concerns for safety and help the survivor develop a realistic safety plan.

- Always provide accurate information about services and facilities.

- Empower the survivor; always allow individuals to make their own choices and decisions.

- Encourage re-engagement in a daily routine and in activities with family and supports within the community.

- Discourage comfort in alcohol or other substance abuse.

Community-Level Support

Community-based activities have been shown to be effective in helping to decrease trauma for GBV survivors. Supportive interventions on the community level include: a) identifying and training traditional, community-based support workers; b) developing women's support groups or support groups specifically designed for survivors of sexual violence and their families; and c) creating special drop-in centers for survivors where they can receive confidential and compassionate attention.

Children & Adolescents

Children and youth are especially vulnerable to GBV given their level of dependence, limited capacity to protect themselves, and limited power and participation in decision-making processes. Health personnel assisting children should have the appropriate level of training and skills. Age appropriate language and creative communication methods should be used (e.g. drawing, games, story-telling). Never coerce or restrain abused children and include trusted family members in the treatment process. Children should not be removed from family care for treatment unless there is abuse or neglect and protection is required.

Regarding adolescents, females may be specifically targeted for sexual violence in situations of armed conflict and severe economic hardship. Health care providers, relief workers and protection officers should devote special attention to their psychosocial needs.

Other Issues

GBV & Domestic Violence

Be cautious in situations where violence has occurred by a spouse or other family member (domestic violence). The survivor and/ or other relatives may be susceptible to further danger and retaliation, especially if the abuser is aware that the incident has been reported. Assess each case on an individual basis, utilizing the support of other colleagues in deciding an appropriate response. Health care providers may choose to refer the matter to a disciplinary committee, inform the authorities, or provide discreet advice to the survivor about the potential options.

Children of Rape

Children born as a result of rape are susceptible to stigma, abuse and even abandonment. Therefore, these children must be monitored closely. Families and mothers particularly should be offered education and support. Foster placement and, later, adoption should be considered if the child is rejected, neglected or abused in other ways.

HIV/AIDS & MENTAL HEALTH

HIV/AIDS Global Summary

Worldwide, an estimated 34 million people were living with HIV at the end of 2010. In 2010, there were 2.7 million new HIV infections. Most newly infected people live in Sub-Saharan Africa and the annual number of newly infected individuals continues to decline. In 2010, an estimated 1.9 million people became infected representing a 16% decrease from the estimated 2.2 million newly infected in 2001. However in regions including the Middle east and North Africa, the annual number of people newly infected with HIV has increased to 59,000 in 2010 compared to 43,000 in 2001. In addition, since 2008, the incidence of HIV infection has grown in Eastern Europe and Central Asia.

Globally, the annual number of people dying from AIDS-related causes continues to decline with an estimated 1.8 million in 2010 compared to 2.2 million in 2005. The number of people dying annually from AIDS-related causes began to decline in 2005 and continues to decrease in sub-Saharan Africa, the Caribbean, and South and Southeast Asia. Unfortunately, AIDS-related deaths have increased dramatically in Central Asia, East Asia, Eastern Europe, the Middle East, and North Africa

The availability of antiretroviral therapy in low– and middle-income countries worldwide (particularly countries in Sub-Saharan Africa) has been responsible for preventing 2.5 million deaths since 1995. Since 1995, more than 350,000 children (86% from Sub-Saharan Africa), have been spared from contracting HIV due to antiretroviral prophylaxis being available to pregnant women living with the virus.

143

New evidence-based studies have indicated also that people living with the HIV are less likely to transmit the virus and that individuals who are HIV-negative and have taken antiretroviral pre-exposure prophylaxis orally as a tablet or vaginally in gel form have reduced their risk of contracting the virus.

HIV/AIDS & Mental Health –General Overview

HIV disease has the capacity to affect the physical, psychological, and social well-being of individuals. A number of the medical diseases associated with HIV manifest as neurological or neuropsychiaric illnesses (e.g. neuropathy, central nervous system infections and tumors). People infected by the virus may be burdened also by emotions such as fear, anger, and guilt, which, if not placed in perspective, may contribute to more severe psychiatric conditions. In addition, social consequences of HIV disease have included stigma, loss of household income and financial stability, and the destruction of family and community structures.

Mental health support in general (e.g. psychoeducation; supportive group, family, and individual counseling; and, in the case of severe illness, medication therapy) may play a role in influencing the overall health of individuals whose lives have been affected by the epidemic. Special forms of counseling, such as HIV information/prevention counseling and adherence counseling, are associated with mental health and are important to decreasing the spread of infection and the proliferation of disease.

Medical Aspects of HIV/AIDS

HIV (Human Immunodeficiency Virus) is a type of virus (specifically a retrovirus) that can invade and destroy cells of the immune system. HIV can cause AIDS (or Acquired Immunodeficiency Syndrome) which is a collection of symptoms or medical conditions that indicate immune dysfunction.

HIV can enter the body through blood, semen, vaginal fluid, and breast milk. HIV is most often transmitted through sexual contact or the transfer of contaminated blood (through blood transfusions or intravenous drug abuse). Infants can be infected in the uterus or through breast-feeding when their mothers are infected with HIV.

Data from several countries indicates that the acquisition and transmission of HIV is reduced with abstinence from sexual activity, condom use, decreased sharing of contaminated drug paraphernalia, screened blood products used for transfusions, and the use of antiretroviral medication . Education and HIV testing are the means by which individuals can understand and take action to prevent or manage disease.

145

Measures of Immunity & HIV Infection: CD4+ Immune Cells & Viral Load

CD4+ T lymphocytes (CD4+ T cells) are cells of the immune system that play a role in protecting the body from certain infections. HIV targets CD4+ T cells, disables their normal function, and facilitates a genetic process that leads to proliferation of the virus. CD4+ T cells can be measured through analysis of a blood sample. The US National Institute of Allergy and Infectious Diseases (NIAID) has cited a normal CD4+ T cell count as 800-1200mm3 (other sources have cited a normal range = 500-1500mm3). A low CD4+ T cell count is an indication of impairment of an aspect of the immune system and raises suspicion for HIV disease. Experts have indicated that counts of less than 500mm3 usually mean damage to the immune system, counts less than 200mm3 mean severe damage, and counts less than 50mm3 mean damage of even greater severity. When antiretroviral medications are used CD4+ T cell counts improve.

The viral "load" is a measure of the amount of viral particles in a given blood sample and may be an indication of one's response to treatment and prognosis. The viral load found in blood has been found to accurately reflect the total burden of HIV in the body.

Phases of HIV Infection

HIV should be viewed as a spectrum of disorders ranging from acute (primary) infection with or without an acute retroviral syndrome, to the asymptomatic state, to advanced disease.

A) Acute Primary Infection

Once HIV enters the body, the virus infects a large number of CD4+ T cells and rapidly multiplies, significantly increasing the viral load. Studies have indicated that following primary infection, as many as 50-70% of infected individuals may develop an acute "flu-like" syndrome, also known as acute retroviral syndrome (ARS). This has been estimated to occur 3-6 weeks after infection and may last from 1-4 weeks. Symptoms of ARS may include fever, sweats, fatigue, joint pain, headache, sore throat and enlarged lymph nodes or glands. Some individuals may also experience a skin rash and neuropsychiatric symptoms such confusion, mood changes, and personality changes. As the immune system mounts a response, the viral load declines and the CD4+ T cell count rises and reconstitutes. As the immune response progresses, symptoms of ARS decrease. Most individuals will then enter a period of clinical latency where the virus is less active.

B) Clinical Latency

During this phase, the virus is still present in the body, but is less active. Many individuals do not have any symptoms of HIV infection. The duration of this period can vary greatly among individuals, but the median has been estimated to be 10 years.

C) Advanced Disease - Progression to AIDS

While symptoms of HIV disease may develop during any phase of infection, the extent of illness is generally increased as the CD4+ T cell count declines. More severe complications of infection have been associated with CD4+ T cell counts < 200mm3. AIDS is diagnosed when an HIV-infected individual has one or more opportunistic infections (discussed in the following sections) and has a CD4+ T cell count < 200mm3 (or CD4 percentage <14% according to the US Center for Disease Control classification).

The World Health Organization (WHO) has developed a clinical staging system (outlined below) for resource-constrained settings where extensive laboratory testing may not be readily available. In this system, AIDS is diagnosed based on the clinical symptoms observed upon examination.

WHO HIV/AIDS Clinical Staging System (for Adults & Adolescents)

A. Primary HIV Infection: asymptomatic; Acute retroviral syndrome (ARS).

B. Clinical Stage 1: asymptomatic, persistent generalized lymphadenopathy (in at least two sites, not including inguinal, for longer than 6 months); this stage may last for several years.

C. Clinical Stage 2 (mild symptomatic stage): moderate weight loss (< 10% of total body weight); recurrent respiratory infections (e.g. bronchitis, otitis media, and pharyngitis, sinusitis); skin conditions (e.g. angular cheilitis, fungal nail infections, herpes zoster, papular pruritic eruptions, recurrent oral ulcerations, and seborrheic dermatitis).

D. Clinical Stage 3 (moderate symptomatic stage): severe weight loss (>10 % of total body weight); unexplained diarrhea > 1 month; pulmonary tuberculosis; severe bacterial infections including pneumonia, pyelonephritis, empyema, pyomyositis, meningitis, bone and joint infections, and bacteremia; other conditions including recurrent oral candidiasis, oral hairy leukoplakia, and acute necrotizing ulcerative stomatitis, gingivitis, or periodontitis.

E. Clinical Stage 4 (severe symptomatic stage): HIV wasting syndrome, HIV encephalopathy, and varied conditions associated with opportunistic infections and tumors related to HIV/AIDS (see next section).

Opportunistic Infections (OIs)

The term opportunistic indicates an infection that takes the "opportunity" to flourish when there is compromised function of the immune system. OIs include Toxoplama encephalitis, cryptococcus, cytomegalovirus, Pneumocytis carinii pneumonia (PCP), Mycobacterium avium complex (MAC), Mycobacterium tuberculosis, herpes simplex, and cryptosporidosis. The causes, locations, symptoms and treatments for some of these conditions are outlined in the table on the next page.

149

III: Conditions & Issues: HIV/AIDS & Mental Health

Opportunistic Infections (OIs) Associated with HIV/AIDS

Name of Opportunistic Infection (OI)	Agent causing Infection	Site of Infection	Symptoms (Sx)	Treatment
Candida albicans	fungus	Mouth/throat, esophagus; vagina	Mouth: white patches on gums, tongue or lining of the mouth; pain; difficulty swallowing; loss of appetite. Vagina: itching, burning, thick, white discharge	Anti-fungal medication
Cryptococcus neoformans	fungus	brain (meninges)	headache, fever	Antifungal medication
Cryptosporidium	parasite	gastrointestinal tract	significant diarrhea	no direct treatment for the parasite; ARV
Cytomegalovirus (CMV)	virus (herpes family)	eyes, nervous system, intestines	Inflammation of the retina, nerves, brain issue, esophagus and bowels	Anti-viral medication
Herpes Simplex (HSV)	virus (alpha herpes sub-family)	mouth, genitals	cold sores/fever blisters; genital sores/lesions	Antiviral medication; there is no cure for HSV though use of antiretrovirals (ARV) may reduce frequency and severity of attacks
Mycobacterium avium complex (MAC) & Mycobacterium tuberculosis (TB)	bacterium	MAC: lungs, lymph glands, liver spleen, blood, bone marrow, intestines, and other organs. TB: lungs, brain, kidneys, or spine.	MAC: constitutional sx; will depend on organs involved (diarrhea, sx of hepatitis, pneumonia; lymphadenopathy; impaired blood count). Latent TB: no symptoms; active TB: cough, night sweats, fever, weight loss, chills, and fatigue.	MAC: antimycobacterial medication course; special precautions to prevent spread of infection. TB: long-term antimycobacterial medication course (beware of liver damage); special precautions to prevent spread of infection.
Pneumocystis Jirovecii (Carinii)	parasite	lungs	dry cough, shortness of breath, fever	Antiparasitic medication
Toxolasma gondii	parasite	brain	Inflamed brain tissue causing headache, fever, weakness in an arm or leg; seizure may also occur	Anti-parasitic medication

Tumors associated with HIV/AIDS

Tumors associated with HIV/AIDS include Kaposi's Sarcoma and Primary Central Nervous System (CNS) Lymphoma. The causes, locations, symptoms and treatments for these conditions are outlined in the table below.

Tumors associated with HIV/AIDS

Tumor Name	Cause	Site of Tumor	Symptoms (Sx)	Treatment
Kaposi's Sarcoma	tumor of the blood vessels	skin most commonly; also lungs, brain, liver, mouth	Skin: painless, purple/black lesions; Lungs: shortness of breath, productive cough/sputum; Brain: seizures; liver dysfunction	depending on area affected cosmetic treatment; chemotherapy or radiation therapy for more extensive disease
Primary Central Nervous System (CNS) Lymphoma	tumor of lymph cells	brain	focal neurological signs depending on location of lesions	radiation and chemotherapy

Medication Therapy For HIV

Significant advances in antiretroviral therapy have been made since the advent of the first US government-approved medication in 1987, zidovudine (AZT). With the development of highly active antiretroviral therapy (HAART), HIV-1 infection has become a chronic, manageable disease for individuals with stable suppression of the virus and access to treatment. HAART is the combination of several antiretroviral medicines used to slow the rate at which HIV multiplies in the body. A combination of three or more antiretroviral medicines (often referred to as a "cocktail") is more effective than using just one medicine (monotherapy) to treat the virus. The current recommendation for starting HAART in the United States is to begin therapy when the CD4+ T cell count falls to 500cells/ml or below. There are sources that have also indicated that, in mid– and low income countries, initiation of therapy is recommended for a CD4+ T cell count of 350cells/ml or below.

Anti-retroviral medications generally target or interfere with steps in the reproductive cycle of the virus. There are 6 classes of anti-retroviral medications currently available:

1) Nucleoside Reverse Transcriptase Inhibitors (NRTIs)

2) Non-Nucleoside Reverse Transcriptase Inhibitors (NNRTIs)

3) Protease Inhibitors (PIs)

4) Integrase Inhibitors (IIs)

5) Fusion Inhibitors (FIs)

6) Chemokine Receptor Antagonists (CRAs).

The use of these medications depends on a variety of factors including simplicity or complexity of use, efficacy determined by clinical evidence, side-effect profile, practice guidelines, and clinician preference. Particular concerns that play a role in which medications are initiated or used for maintenance therapy include adverse effects, co-infection with hepatitis B virus or hepatitis C virus, pregnancy, and resistance. Outlined below and on subsequent pages are lists of antiretroviral medications currently in use.

Nucleoside Reverse Transcriptase Inhibitors (NRTI)

Abacavir (Ziagen)

Didanosine (Videx)

Emtricitabine (Emtriva)

Lamivudine (Epivir)

Stavudine (Zerit)

Tenofovir (Viread)

Zidovudine (Retrovir)

Non-Nucleoside Reverse Transcriptase Inhibitors (NNRTI)

Delavirdine (Rescriptor)

Efavirenz (Sustiva)

Nevirapine (Viramune, Viramune XR)

Rilpivirine (Edurant)

Protease Inhibitors (PI)

Atazanavir (Reyataz)

Darunavir (Prezista)

Fosamprenavir (Lexiva)

Indinavir (Crixivan)

Lopinavir/Ritonavir (Kaletra)

Nelfinavir (Viracept)

Ritonavir (Norvir)

Saquinavir (Invirase)

Tipranavir (Aptivus)

III: Conditions & Issues: HIV/AIDS & Mental Health

Integrase Inhibitor (II)

Raltegravir (Isentress)

Chemokine Receptor Antagonist (CRA)

Maraviroc (Selzentry)

Fusion Inhibitor (FI)

Enfuvirtide (Fuzeon)

Combination Formulations

Atripla - Tenofovir + emtricitabine + efavirenz

Combivir - Zidovudine + lamivudine

Complera – Tenofovir + emtricitabine + rilpivirine

Epzicom - Abacavir + lamivudine

Stribild – elvitegravir + cobicistat + emtricitabine + tenofovir

Trizivir - Abacavir + lamivudine + zidovudine

Truvada - Tenofovir + emtricitabine

III: Conditions & Issues: HIV/AIDS & Mental Health

While antiretroviral therapy can help control proliferation of the virus and allow the body to recover its ability to fight infections, it is not a cure. If anti-retroviral therapy is discontinued, the virus will recur. Other reasons for treatment failure may include drugs or herbal preparations that interfere and reduce the level of antiretroviral medication in the system; a patient's being too ill (i.e. overwhelmed by not only HIV infection but also other infections or illnesses); an individual's inability to tolerate the medicine (e.g. due to significant side effects); resistance; or poor adherence to the prescribed medications.

Resistance

HIV makes every effort to survive in the body. If there is anti-retroviral medication in the system but not at a level to effectively disable the virus, the virus can potentially mutate or change to a form that can resist the effects of the medication. This capacity to change and resist medication effects is termed **resistance.** Resistance is an important reason why HIV drugs stop working. Missed doses of medication or continuing on a drug regimen that is not effective can encourage resistance. Interactions with other medicines that reduce HIV medication in the system or a poor ability to absorb HIV medication into the bloodstream can also contribute to resistance.

Adherence

The risk of resistance may be reduced by maintaining adherence to the anti-retroviral medicines prescribed. Adherence, in simple terms, means the ability to take medications as prescribed. Specifically, adherence involves a) taking the appropriate anti-retroviral drugs; b) taking the drugs on the appropriate schedule; and c) taking the drugs in the correct manner (e.g. with or without food). One hundred percent adherence is required for treatment to be effective. With precise adherence, antiretroviral therapy will be successful. With poor adherence continued viral replication and increased viral load may occur, the CD4+ T cell count may decrease (increasing the risk for opportunistic infections), and the potential for resistance may emerge. It can be challenging for individuals to maintain 100% adherence. Adherence counselling provides those with difficulty support and techniques to improve and maintain adherence. Specific techniques are outlined in a subsequent section of this chapter.

HIV & Sexually Transmitted Diseases (STDs)

Sexually transmitted diseases (STDs) are infections that are passed from one individual to another through sexual contact. The infections may be caused by varied pathogens such as viruses (e.g. HIV, hepatitis) or bacteria (e.g. syphilis, gonorrhea). STDs may increase a person's risk for becoming infected with HIV by causing conditions that allow easier passage of the virus into the body (e.g. passage through open sores, ulcers, and irritations). The inflammatory process (resulting from damage by certain STDs to the skin surface) increases the presence and concentration of immune cells to the area that can serve as targets for HIV (e.g. CD4+ cells). In addition, those infected with HIV, who contract subsequent STDs, are at increased risk of transmitting the virus to sexual partners. Studies indicate that those infected with HIV and also have other STDs can shed the virus in their genital secretions. The higher the concentration of HIV in genital fluids, the more likely the virus may be spread to a partner.

Contracting an STD may have serious implications for one who is HIV-positive. Some STDs are curable or eradicated with antibiotic treatment (e.g. gonorrhea, syphilis). However, others may not be eradicated fully and may be associated with potentially fatal diseases such as cancer (HPV, Hep C) and liver failure (Hep B, Hep C). The table on the next page outlines a number of STDs that have been associated with HIV.

Sexually Transmitted Diseases (STDs) Associated With HIV

Bacterial

Syphilis

Gonorrhea

Chlamydia

Trichomoniasis

Viral

Hepatitis A (Hep A)

Hepatitis B (Hep B)

Hepatitis C (Hep C)

Herpes Simplex Virus (HSV)

Human Papilloma Virus (HPV)

Psychiatric Conditions & Psychosocial Issues Associated with HIV/AIDS

1. Psychiatric Conditions

HIV-related medical conditions causing psychiatric symptoms

a) HIV-related dementia

Dementia is defined generally as a mental disorder causing impaired intellectual functioning (e.g. ability to reason), impaired memory and orientation, distractibility, changes in mood and personality, and impaired judgment. Dementia may be caused by varied conditions such as degenerative brain diseases (e.g. Alzheimer's Disease), vascular (blood vessel) disease, or chronic alcohol or drug abuse. The onset of dementia is typically insidious or slow lasting months to years. Dementias that involve ongoing degeneration or destruction of brain tissue are usually irreversible.

HIV may directly damage brain tissue leading to a dementia-like syndrome. Over the years, several names have been attached to more severe and milder aspects of HIV-related dementia and have included AIDS dementia complex (ADC), HIV associated dementia (HAD), HIV-encephalopathy, subacute encephalitis, HIV cognitive/motor complex (HIV CMC), minor cognitive-motor disorder, and HIV associated neurocognitive disease (HAND).

The dementia associated with HIV can develop over weeks or chronically over years. Symptoms may be similar to those associated with other types of dementia and include decreased short-term memory, decreased attention and concentration, disturbance in word finding, decelerated thought processing, psychomotor retardation (i.e. slowed movement), impaired reasoning and intellect, and, in advanced disease, impaired visual-spatial function (i.e. aspect of brain function that analyzes and understands space in two and three dimensions). Personality changes and mood disturbances such as depression may occur. Less commonly, manic symptoms (agitation, irritability, impulsivity, and excessive talkativeness) and psychosis (hallucinations, delusions, irrational suspiciousness, or paranoia) may be present. Motor deficits (i.e. impaired movement) are also a part of the HIV-related dementia syndrome and may include muscle weakness, increased or decreased muscle tone, spasticity movements, muscle rigidity or "cogwheeling," and over or under- reactive reflexes.

A complete medical and psychiatric evaluation are important in evaluating an individual with HIV who presents with neurocognitive symptoms. Where available, laboratory tests (e.g. complete blood count, CD4 count, HIV viral load, chemistry screen, urinalysis, blood/urine cultures, ECG, chest x-ray, and, when applicable, drug toxicology screen, thyroid function tests, and B6 & B12 vitamin levels) and neuroimaging (e.g. magnetic resonance imaging or MRI) are used in the evaluation of HIV-related dementia.

HIV-related dementia has been treatable. That is, symptoms may be reduced with anti-retroviral therapy. Specific psychiatric symptoms of the dementia syndrome may be addressed with particular treatments as well. For example, if agitation has developed and is severe, low dose antipsychotic may be used (e.g. olanzapine or seroquel if available or chlorpromazine). Low dose antipsychotics may be used if hallucinations are present as well. Avoiding antipsychotics causing extrapyramidal symptoms (EPS) is generally recommended.

Use of antipsychotics in elderly individuals for psychosis related to other (non HIV-related) dementias has not been recommended due to increased risk of death. Caution is also taken with elderly people with HIV-related dementia. Antidepressants are helpful in treating associated depression. Benzodiazepines that are metabolized by the body in a relatively short period (i.e. those with short half-lives such as lorazepam) may be useful for anxiety and insomnia. However, it is important to be aware that benzodiazepines have also been associated with uninhibited behavior (i.e. disinhibition) and cognitive impairment. They should be used short-term and in the lowest effective doses.

b) CNS infections and tumors

Individuals with significant HIV disease may be prone to central nervous system (CNS) infections and tumors that can present with a combination of neurological and psychiatric symptoms. These conditions are outlined in detail below and include neurosyphilis, cryptococcal meningitis, toxoplasmosis, cytomegalovirus (CMV) encephalitis, aseptic meningitis, progressive multifocal leukoencephalopathy (PML), and CNS lymphoma.

Neurosyphilis

Syphilis is an infection caused by the spirochete, Treponema pallidum, and has several stages of disease. The primary stage is characterized by enlarged lymph nodes in the groin region and a painless "chancre" or sore that may be located on the genitals. This may disappear without treatment but secondary syphilis characterized by fever, swollen lymph nodes, rash, and genital lesions may appear after approximately 2 years. During this stage a syphilitic meningitis with headache, nausea, stiff neck, and occasional cranial nerve deficits, may occur. However, more commonly, there are no neurological symptoms but diagnostic tests analyzing spinal fluid may be abnormal. The latent or next phase is also characterized by abnormal diagnostic blood tests and minimal clinical symptoms.

The last stage or tertiary phase is when neurosyphilis (syphilis affecting brain tissue) occurs. During this phase other organs including the heart and eyes my be affected as well. Neurosyphilis may present with or without symptoms , however diagnostic tests (of spinal fluid) remain abnormal. Syphilis in this stage may cause meningitis or a stroke. There may also be syphilitic dementia associated with seizures, mania, agitation, and grandiose delusional thoughts. Tabes dorsalis (ataxia/loss of balance, lower extremity paresthesia and paresis, hyporeflexia, incontinence, and sharp pains) may occur. "Gummas" or degenerated brain tissue surrounded by thick, fiber-like tissue may, on rare occasion, lead to a space-occupying brain mass.

Syphilis may be suspected or detected through tests including VDRL (Venereal Disease Research Laboratory), RPR (rapid plasma reagent), MH-ATP (microhemiagglutination – assay for treponema pallidum), and FTA (fluorescent treponemal antibody). In some instances lumbar puncture may be indicated. Treatment with antibiotics is effective.

Cryptococcal Meningitis

Cryptococcus neoformans is a fungus that commonly causes meningitis (swelling of the protective outer-sheath of the brain) in AIDS patients. Symptoms may occur within days or weeks. Early symptoms may be fever, lethargy, persistent, progressive headache; seizure and delirium may occur. Stiff neck typically associated with other types of meningitis is not neces-sarily present. Some individuals may develop focal neurological symptoms including paralysis of cranial nerves causing blindness and deafness, partial muscle weakness, and over-active reflexes.

Treated or untreated, the disease may progress to produce complications including seizure, stroke, swelling of the brain, and coma. Permanent nerve damage and dementia may be long-lasting complications. Cryptococcus is detected usually by analyzing blood and spinal fluid for presence of the fun-gus. Antifungal antibiotics are used as treatment.

164

Toxoplasmosis

Toxoplasmosis is an infection caused by the parasite, Toxoplasma gondii. It is characterized by multiple abcesses that cause swelling of brain tissue or encephalitis.

Initial symptoms may include enlarged lymph nodes in the neck and flu-like symptoms such as headache, fever, malaise. Localized neurological signs may be present and include partial muscle weakness, partial loss of sensation, partial loss of sight, inability to comprehend or communicate speech, memory loss, and seizure. Delirium may develop with disease progression. Nausea, vomiting, and lethargy may be an indication of increased pressure within the skull as the brain tissue continually inflames.

If available, a computerized tomography (CT) or magnetic resonance imaging (MRI) scan may reveal the presence of the disease (ring-enhancing lesions). Anti-parasitic medication has been an effective treatment.

Cytomegalovirus (CMV) Encephalitis

CMV belongs to the family of Herpes viruses and in addition to neurological disease is associated with disease of the eyes, lungs, esophagus, intestines, and adrenal gland. Neuropsychiatric manifestations of CMV include primarily encephalitis (global swelling or inflammation of brain tissue). Symptoms associated with encephalitis include fever, headache, lethargy, delirium, dementia, seizure, and coma. Occasionally facial and ocular cranial nerve impairments, and weakness of the lower limbs occurs. A definitive diagnosis is made through brain biopsy (analysis of a sample of brain tissue). The recommended treatment is antiviral medication.

Aseptic Meningitis

A form of meningitis may occur where no pathogen or germ is evident on diagnostic analysis (i.e. no bacteria evident in spinal fluid). This has been referred to as aseptic meningitis. Symptoms may emerge within days to weeks and include headache with or without stiff neck or fever, lethargy and delirium. Rarely impairment of the cranial nerve that controls movements of the facial muscles occurs.

If available, a CT or MRI will indicate inflammation of the tissues that make up a protective sheath enveloping the brain (meninges) and analysis of the spinal fluid will be abnormal.

There is no specific treatment – however the condition may resolve on its own. Supportive measures (e.g. IV fluid), antiretroviral therapy, pain medication, and steroids are used empirically.

Progressive Multifocal Leukoencephalopathy (PML)

PML is caused by a virus (John Cunningham or JC virus) that infects and destroys oligodendrocytes (i.e. CNS cells that produce a protective cover that aids the transmission of nervous impulses from one nerve cell to another) and other supportive cells (astrocytes). Neurological and psychiatric symptoms have included impaired cognition (e.g. memory and concentration), weakness and sensory loss, impaired vision, slurred speech, loss of muscle coordination, dizziness, seizures, inability to understand or communicate speech, inability to read, and inability to recognize faces.

If available, an MRI is preferred to CT as lesions in white matter of the brain will be more evident. The prognosis for PML is poor although some antiretroviral medications have been associated with prolonged life.

Primary CNS Lymphoma

Central nervous system (CNS) lymphoma associated with AIDS occurs most commonly when there is severe immunodeficiency. Symptoms include headache, seizure, lethargy, and delirium. Focal or localized neurological signs are not uncommon and may include impaired capacity to understand or communicate speech, muscle weakness, and cranial nerve deficits. If available, a CT or MRI scan may reveal one or more homogenous, mass lesions. Treatment involves radiation, steroids, and/or chemotherapy.

c) Other Medical Conditions & Medications

Other medical conditions seen in HIV-infected individuals causing psychiatric symptoms have included kidney disease (HIV-associated nephropathy and end -stage renal disease), liver disease (hepatitis C, cirrhosis), and endocrine disorders (hypothyroidism, diabetes mellitus, hypotestosteronism, and adrenal insufficiency). Antiretroviral therapy (ART) can be toxic and cause neurobehavioral disturbances. In particular, efavirenz has been associated with cognitive changes, headache, dizziness, insomnia, nightmares, and even suicidal thought. Symptoms appear to be related to blood levels and tend to decrease gradually over time, however. HIV-infected individuals who are taking interferon for treatment of coinfection with the hepatitis C virus (HCV) may be at risk for depression. Antidepressant medication is indicated if depressive symptoms are persistent and debilitating.

Psychiatric Illnesses Associated with HIV/AIDS

According to western studies (United States), psychiatric illnesses occurring commonly in individuals with HIV or AIDS include depression, anxiety disorders, adjustment disorder, and substance abuse. With certain conditions, mania and psychosis have also been observed.

Studies from the United States have indicated that depression and suicidal thoughts and attempts may be increased in people infected with HIV. Risk factors for suicide have included a recently positive HIV test, having lost close friends to AIDS, poor social and financial support, continuous relapses of medical illnesses associated with HIV, and the presence of dementia or delirium.

According to American studies, anxiety disorders that occur with frequency in individuals with HIV have included generalized anxiety disorder, post-traumatic stress disorder, and obsessive-compulsive disorder. An adjustment disorder, according to the DSM V, is characterized by emotional or behavioral distress occurring in response to an identifiable stressor within 3 months of the stressor. Adjustment disorder with anxiety or depressive features has been associated with HIV and AIDS.

Substance abuse may play a role in putting individuals at risk for contracting HIV or may occur as a means of self-medicating distress after infection has been realized. Intravenous drug abuse or sharing contaminated drug paraphernalia remains a significant mode of HIV transmission throughout the world. People who abuse substances are at risk for engaging in unsafe sexual practices which contributes to the spread of the disease. People with HIV who do not have access to mental health services may abuse substances in order to cope with stress, further complicating or perpetuating HIV disease and emotional distress.

Studies have indicated that mania has been associated with opportunistic infections (e.g. cryptococcal meningitis) and medications (e.g. efavirnez). In addition, it has occured as an aspect of HIV-associated dementia. For those with a pre-existing bipolar disorder, an exacerbation of symptoms tends to occur most commonly, but not exclusively, in the context of HIV-associated dementia. Psychotic symptoms (e.g. hallucinations) have been observed as an aspect of HIV-associated dementia .

The specific symptoms and treatments for depression, anxiety disorders, adjustment disorder, substance abuse, and mania are outlined in previous chapters. Regarding psychiatric medication therapy, drugs that are less likely to interfere with or potentiate the side effects of anti-retroviral medicines are recommended.

2. Psychological Issues

Common Emotions

Fear, uncertainty, anger, and guilt are emotions often experienced by individuals infected by HIV.

Individuals may be fearful and uncertain about the effect the virus will have on their bodies and their lives in general. They may fear subsequent medical tests, losing the capacity to function at full strength, and losing the support of friends and family. Providing them education and information can reduce fear and uncertainty. For example, directly teaching or referring individuals to healthcare providers who can educate them about test procedures, medications, and recognizing symptoms of illness early can help them feel in greater control of their circumstances. In addition helping them identify reliable supports (family, friends, clergy, therapist, etc...) can allay fears of abandonment.

Anger is common and may be rooted in a sense of unfairness. That is, an individual may feel that he or she has been unduly afflicted. Anger may also stem from a fear of losing control of one's life or a fear of social stigma, rejection, or abandonment. It will be important to help the patient understand that having anger is alright and a natural human response. The issue is how the anger is managed. Helping the individual identify and utilize constructive, productive ways to discharge anger is imperative.

Guilt is another emotion that is often experienced by individuals infected with HIV. A person with HIV may feel that he or she has brought the virus onto him or herself and should be blamed and punished. Some experience guilt about introducing HIV into the lives of others. They may feel that they have created burden and distress for spouses, partners, parents, children, or friends. Individuals burdened with overwhelming guilt, should be counseled on how to detach negativity and punishment from the virus. Help them understand that, in reality, the virus has nothing to do with punishment. Anyone, "good" or "bad," has the potential to become infected. In addition, reinforce patients' self esteem and sense of worth. Having the patients remind themselves of who they are outside of having HIV can bolster self confidence and esteem. Having them recall what people who love them (i.e. family, partners, friends) like about them can reinforce self esteem.

Loss of control

With the advent of Highly Active Antiretroviral Therapy (HAART), people with HIV are living longer and may be less severely debilitated by disease. HAART may contribute to one's maintaining a sense of independence and control over his or her life. Emphasizing one's capacity to function and providing reassurance and reinforcement of function can help individuals living with HIV preserve self-esteem and self-worth.

Caregivers should allow patients to take the lead in expressing what feels like too much or too little help. Those caring for individuals with HIV disease may find it useful to listen without necessarily providing advice to resolve a problem. Attending to non-verbal clues and keeping an open channel of communication can be useful.

Newly Diagnosed Individuals

Reactions will vary among people newly diagnosed with HIV. It will be important to help the individual identify support that suits his or her individual needs (e.g. some utilize family, friends, mental health professionals, literature about HIV disease, or spiritual resources). In addition, providing factual, practical information will help dispel fear and uncertainty. Assessing the patient's level of comfort with disclosing his or her HIV status and the need to make previous partners aware is important.

Death & Dying

Despite the advances in treatment, in some areas of the world, HIV/AIDS still remains a serious disease from which individuals may die.

Emotional responses to death and dying, including denial, anger, bargaining, depression, and acceptance, have been described by Kubler-Ross and are outlined in detail in the chapter on "Loss & Bereavement." These emotions are not necessarily experienced by patients in a particular sequence and caregivers may also experience these reactions. Helping both patients and caregivers accept the limitations on what they can do or control within the situation is important. Helping individuals identify and focus on the positives and reframe negative thoughts can be useful. Patients and caregivers should be encouraged to identify and actively incorporate into their lives those things that give them pleasure.

173

3. Social Issues

Women & HIV/AIDS

HIV and AIDS in women can significantly impact households and societies. In many developing countries, women are the primary caregivers of the family. When the mother becomes ill, young daughters are often pulled from school, forfeiting an education to help in the home. In some cultures, if a woman loses her husband she may be at risk of losing land or property. Faced with such a challenge, some women have been driven to prostitution in exchange for food or other goods.

Social stigma

Social stigma is common in many societies and can interfere with family and community support for individuals contracting disease. Individuals with HIV or AIDS have the burden of being rejected by family and friends and may even be accused of "contaminating' or tainting a family's name.

Poverty

In countries that are already poverty stricken, the AIDS epidemic may cause households an even greater decline into complete destitution. Households that are already impoverished may have difficulty overcoming additional adversity. AIDS may cause the loss of productive household members resulting in loss of income.

Decreased income means less ability to feed, cloth, or educate family members. In some instances families separate and children may be forced to start working early to support the family.

High Medical Costs

The high medical costs associated with HIV and AIDS treatment can potentially devastate families and individuals in both developed and developing countries. For example, in the United States, people with HIV/AIDS without insurance or other financial resources may be unable to access adequate care. There are limitations on support for the indigent. Even for those who have some form of health insurance, the high cost of medical services and medications are not always adequately covered. Despite increases in funding for HIV/AIDS in recent years, many developing countries continue to have limited access to services and medications.

Specialized Counseling Associated With HIV/AIDS

HIV voluntary counseling & testing (VCT)

a. HIV counseling

The aim of HIV counseling is to decrease the acquisition and transmission of HIV through providing effective *information* and *prevention counseling* .

Information

It is suggested that all who are recommended or request HIV testing receive information that includes the risk factors for transmission; how to prevent transmission; benefits of getting tested; the consequences of not testing if one is at risk; importance of and explicit instructions on how to obtain test results; the meaning or interpretation of results; how and where to obtain additional information about HIV; and how and where to obtain additional services if indicated (e.g. medical, psychological, social services).

Information should always be provided in a manner that is appropriate to culture, language, age, and developmental level. While face-to-face, client-counselor sessions are recommended for prevention counseling, pamphlets or videos are appropriate (and an efficient means) for providing information about HIV.

Prevention counseling

There have been a number of proficient models for HIV prevention counseling. The client-centered HIV prevention counseling approach has been shown to be both efficient and effective. Client-centered counseling focuses on the client's own unique situation and involves helping the client outline and achieve an explicit behavior change goal to decrease the chance of acquiring or transmitting HIV. For individuals taking the standard HIV test, the client-centered approach involves two brief, in-person or face-to-face sessions with a health provider or counselor. In the first session, an assessment of the client's personal HIV risk is made; a risk behavior (if any) and action to change that behavior is identified and discussed; the HIV test is performed; and the client is asked to return in 2 weeks for results.

In the second session, progress made in changing the previously identified risk behavior is discussed, additional behavior change actions are outlined as needed, HIV test results are provided and discussed, and referral to additional services is offered as indicated.

With rapid testing, there may be either one or two sessions depending on test results. Individuals with preliminary positive rapid HIV test results will have another session when they return for their confirmatory results. Clients at risk for HIV but with negative rapid HIV test results receive one session of counseling that includes a risk-reduction plan. While not obligated to return, they should be offered the opportunity to come back for a follow-up session to discuss their efforts to implement the plan.

Client-centered HIV Prevention Counseling – Session #1

1st SESSION

1. Assess the client's <u>personal risk</u> for HIV. *What in particular puts this individual at risk for HIV?* Ask in a non-judgmental way and use active, attentive listening to determine whether the client engages in risk behaviors such as unprotected sex with others who may be at risk for HIV; abuse of intravenous drugs or other mind-altering substances that could alter judgment or has had blood transfusions or exposure to contaminated blood products. Risk also involves one's maintaining misconceptions such as the belief that he or she could never be afflicted or that their culture or society could never understand or accept using precautions against HIV. It is important to help the client identify and understand these "risks" as well. Discuss in a sensitive manner the circumstances that put them at risk. Remember that this is not the time to discuss the meaning of test results (this is covered at another point in the counseling process). Also, the counselor should not engage in discussions of additional problems unrelated to the client's specific HIV risk factors (discussing other illnesses, social problems, etc…). There will be another time in the counseling process to address these issues as well.

2. Explore attempts already made to reduce risk behaviors. If the client already engaged in risk-reducing behavior, acknowledge his or her success. Also, encourage discussion of the challenges that made decreasing risk behavior difficult and discuss how these challenges were managed.

3. If there is an identifiable risk factor (e.g. unprotected sex) and action has not been taken already to decrease the risky behavior, discuss a *specific, concrete action* that can help reduce the risk (e.g. provide information on the proper use of and how to obtain condoms and ask the client to use them between now and the time he returns for the HIV test results).

4. Describe, discuss, and answer questions regarding the HIV testing process.

Client-centered HIV Prevention Counseling – Session #2

2nd SESSION

---

1. Discuss the progress made in changing the previously identified risk behavior.

2. Identify additional risk behaviors and outline concrete actions to change the behaviors (as indicated).

3. Provide and discuss the meaning of the HIV test results (see the section on the next page on "HIV Testing").

Offer referral to additional services, as indicated (i.e. medical, psychological, social).

b. HIV testing

The HIV test is designed to detect antibodies to the virus. A confirmed positive test result indicates that antibodies are present and that HIV infection has occurred. Test kits used currently have the capacity to screen varied body fluids including blood products (whole blood, serum, and plasma), oral fluid, and urine (see the table on the next page). Factors influencing the type of test kit used by a health facility may include the ease of sample collection, cost, accuracy or sensitivity of the test, client preferences and acceptability, and the likelihood of clients returning for results.

HIV Tests and Their Properties

Test Type	Type of Body Fluid Collected	Availability of Preliminary Test Results (time frame)	Comments
Standard HIV Test Enzyme Immuno-Assay (EIA) Test	Blood (serum, plasma) via phle-botomy	2 weeks; results obtained in person	High accuracy or sensitivity; easy to process a large number of tests in a short time frame; client must return for test result increasing the potential for no return
Oral Fluid Test (EIA)	Fluid from surface of tissues within the mouth	2 weeks; results obtained in person	Noninvasive sample collection decreasing potential for spread of infection
Urine Test (EIA)	Urine via urine cup	2 weeks; results obtained in person	Noninvasive sample collection decreasing potential for spread of infection
Home Sample Collection Test	Dried blood drop via finger stick and sample is sent to a lab for analysis	3 – 7 days; results obtained by tele-phone	Convenient; greater privacy and anonymity; less invasive sample collection
Rapid Test	Blood (serum, plasma) via phle-botomy or less invasive finger stick	10 – 20 minutes; results obtained in person	Convenient; less invasive sample collection; client is already present for result (chance for no return for results is di-minished)
Ora-Quick (oral in-home HIV test)	Fluid from surface of tissues within the mouth	20-40 minutes	Available over-the-counter
Polymerase Chain Reaction (PCR) Test	Blood	3-7 days	Used to test blood supplies or babies born to HIV positive mothers; expensive

181

Positive HIV Test Results

If an initial HIV test result is positive, additional confirmatory tests are done to verify the result (i.e. Western Blot Test with results available in 2 weeks). An HIV test is considered positive only after both the initial and confirmatory tests are positive. A confirmed positive test is an indication that HIV infection has occurred.

Negative HIV Test Results

A negative HIV test result strongly indicates the absence of HIV infection and does not warrant repeating unless there has been new exposure to an infected partner (or partner of unknown HIV status) or exposure to other risk factors (e.g. contaminated drug paraphernalia; working with potentially contaminated blood products or body fluids). An HIV test may be falsely negative if the test was performed prior to seroconversion (i.e. before an individual exposed to virus has developed detectable antibodies to the virus). After exposure to the virus, it may take 4 – 12 weeks before the body develops HIV antibodies that will be detectable by testing. In this situation, individuals should be instructed to repeat the test in 3 months. If the result is negative yet concern still remains (e.g. if one is sure that he or she has had sexual contact with an infected person or contact with contaminated body fluids) another test may be performed 6 months after the exposure.

Adherence Counseling

The ability to take medications as prescribed is termed adherence. One hundred percent adherence is required for antiretroviral medication therapy to be effective. With poor adherence continued viral replication may occur and the CD4+ T cell count may continue to decrease, increasing the risk for opportunistic infections and advanced disease. In addition, non-adherence can lead to resistance (where the HIV changes in character or "mutates" and becomes resistant to a medication's previous effect) resulting in treatment failure. Managing adherence to antiretroviral medication therapy can be a significant challenge for people with HIV disease. Outlined below are a few direct and indirect measures utilized to monitor medication adherence.

Measures of Medication Adherence

- Viral load testing
- Pill counts MEMS (medication event monitoring system) bottle cap
- Self report tools
- One-on-one direct interview by counselor
- Reports from caregivers
- Pharmacy tracking of medication pickup/delivery
- Clinic visits

Adherence counseling involves identifying and addressing *patient, provider, and medication regimen* factors that may contribute to one's difficulty in taking antiretroviral medication as prescribed.

Patient factors contributing to non-adherence

    a) Patient commitment and readiness for treatment.

    b) Social demographics – stability of living situation and work schedule are important factors.

    c) Psychological factors – depression; psychoactive drug abuse may interfere with adherence to antiretroviral medication.

    d) Individual cultural/religious beliefs – beliefs around the need or use of medication may influence adherence.

    e) Physical factors - presence of other medical illnesses.

Management of patient factors :

    a) Evaluate and develop patient's knowledge and understanding of the need for antiretroviral therapy.

    b) Evaluate patient's motivation and commitment to antiretroviral therapy. Peer interventions (interactions with and education from others who are managing HIV disease) have been shown to be effective.

    c) Assess and address mental health issues and behavioral/coping skills with appropriate referrals to support.

Provider factors contributing to non-adherence

a) General support and support when a change in medication therapy is warranted.

b) Patient education.

c) Medication reminders.

d) Use of multidisciplinary team when possible so that care and support can be comprehensive.

e) Ongoing support – studies indicate that adherence diminishes over time when interaction or support from providers is diminished.

f) Access to obstetric and pediatric care as indicated.

Management of provider factors:

a) Providers must offer: education about HIV disease; the need for antiretroviral therapy; the relationship between adherence, resistance, and treatment failure; and significant effects and side effects of medication.

b) Adherence interventions should be offered at the beginning, at points of change, and throughout an established course of therapy.

c) Medication pill boxes, MEMS (medication event monitoring system) bottle caps, alarms, calendars, diaries, phone reminders, and incentive items (gifts) should be utilized as indicated to help patients keep track of their medicines.

d) A multidisciplinary team approach should be utilized to foster a well-rounded view and management of the patient.

Medication regimen factors contributing to non-adherence

   a) individual history and lifestyle which will vary and influence choices of therapy;

   b) dosing frequency;

   c) drug class pill burden; drug interactions and side effects.

Management of medication regimen factors:

a) Evaluation of lifestyle such as eating, sleeping, and work patterns.

b) Evaluating a patient's preferences regarding pill size and number of pills to be taken.

c) Potential for drug interactions and side effects should be carefully assessed.

HIV/AIDS & Disaster/Emergency Settings

Emergency situations such as armed conflicts (war) or natural disasters have the potential to create conditions that make people vulnerable to disease. Challenges within the emergency setting associated with the spread of HIV have included increased economic hardship; disabled health, social and educational services; disabled monitoring and maintenance of blood supply; increased drug abuse; and violent sexual crimes.

Increased Economic Hardship

Economic hardship can increase vulnerability to HIV. In armed conflict situations widows and children left behind may become vulnerable and with little protection. They may become targets of sexual abuse. In addition, women who are left with no means to support themselves, following the loss of family or possessions, may resort to prostitution for survival, potentially increasing the risk of infection.

Disabled Health, Social, & Educational Services

During emergencies people may not be able to receive adequate healthcare because facilities are poorly supplied, have been destroyed, or have closed down. Healthcare personnel may have been lost or internally displaced. Similarly, institutions and personnel used to educate people about HIV/AIDS may be affected.

Disabled Monitoring & Maintenance of Blood Supply

During emergencies, health services may no longer have the capacity to screen blood products adequately and sometimes are forced to recycle existing supplies such as gloves and needles. Although efforts are made to maintain good hygiene and sanitation, the risk for contamination may be increased.

Increased Drug Abuse

In the emergency setting people may become homeless and forced onto the streets where there is greater exposure and access to illicit drugs. Law enforcement services may be disabled making it easier for illegal drugs to be trafficked and sold to greater numbers of people.

Violent Sexual Crimes

Law enforcement agencies may function less efficiently and effectively during emergencies compromising the safety of individuals within communities. In armed conflict situations, women may be at increased risk for being sexually assaulted. Increases in violent crimes such as rape may be seen.

COUNSELING GUIDE

GUIDELINES FOR COUNSELING, COMMUNITY EDUCATION, & COMMUNITY PSYCHOSOCIAL DEVELOPMENT

Counseling—General

Mental health counseling is an important intervention for helping people maintain mental wellness. Counseling is focused on educating, guiding, and referring people in the community to psychological support services as opposed to psychotherapy where professional therapists administer established formal techniques.

Specifically, counseling involves empathic listening, understanding the basic signs of psychological distress, and problem solving skills including basic advice on how to cope with distress, and obtain a more detailed evaluation and treatment if necessary. Counselors also provide individuals, families, and the community with information about mental wellness and raise the public's awareness of stigma and other key mental health issues through community education activities.

Individual Counseling

Counseling for individuals may aim to improve knowledge or to provide an outlet for expressing feelings associated with mental conditions. Basic counseling interventions for individuals are outlined in sections of the manual that discuss specific mental conditions.

Group Counseling

There are many different types of therapeutic groups. People can come together on a variety of shared concerns, issues, and conditions. Some groups require a different approach from other groups (e.g. a group focused on medical issues and their consequences ask for a different approach than a group focused on psychological issues or traumatic experiences). In some groups the group leaders will find some participants who are eager to share their experiences and some who are hesitant to speak. The intellectual and emotional levels of the groups may vary and therefore impact the methods used and program planning. Some groups may be led by professional psychotherapists while others, such as self help groups, are initiated by facilitators with basic group support skills.

Self-help groups

A self-help group is a group of people with similar experiences who meet on a regular basis to help each other to deal with issues related to a health condition or specific experience. People with similar experiences can help each other in the healing process. In self-help groups people can find support, attention, and other participants who can be examples of how to deal with problems. These groups are usually flexible and without a set number of sessions. Participants may attend when they want and facilitation or leadership of the group is less structured. Self help groups may be useful as a single supportive intervention or in combination with other interventions such as individual counseling.

The purpose of self help groups is to provide a means for:

    1) Sharing information and knowledge about a problem;

    2) meeting others who can empathize because of having a similar experience;

    3) support and empowerment;

    4) recognition and acknowledgement;

    5) self expression and making contact;

    6) regaining self confidence;

    7) learning alternative constructive coping methods.

Advantages and ways that self-help groups may differ from professional psychotherapy groups include:

1) Leaders and participants have had similar experiences and both openly share their experiences. There is less potential for power differences between facilitator and group members.

2) Self-help groups may be less expensive (and therefore more accessible) as professional therapists may charge significant fees for their services.

Possible disadvantages of self help groups include:

1) Potential periods where emotional turbulence and conflict between group members is less controlled since there is less structure and professional guidance;

2) No guarantee of continuity since regular attendance is not a set rule and group leadership can change frequently;

3) Screening participants is limited, so there may be difficulty in managing the needs of individuals who have emotional or intellectual capacities that vary significantly from other group members;

4) In acutely stressful situations such as situations of massive loss, people may find that sharing experiences with others amplifies their distress rather than reduces it.

How to lead a self help group

Usually groups are led by two co-leaders who have had experiences similar to other group members and who have been participants in a self help group in the past. The advantage of having two leaders is that they can be a support for one another when difficult issues emerge, the group can continue uninterrupted if one leader must miss a session, and logistical organizational tasks may be shared.

It is important for group leaders to have some basic knowledge of psychological conditions so that additional supportive resources may be offered to individuals who appear to have additional needs. During group sessions it is common for individuals to express strong emotions (e.g. anger) and it is also common for overall themes or attitudes to emerge from the group as a whole (e.g. "scape-goating" - the group appears to "gang up on" or blame a particular member for a conflict or distress that has emerged within the group).

Other common problems that arise in groups include one individual dominating the discussion, individuals selectively withdrawing or refusing to speak, or individuals being excluded from the discussion. It is important that leaders have an awareness and basic knowledge of problematic emotions and themes – sometimes these emotions and themes can be so strong that the group becomes distracted and led astray from the constructive purpose of their gathering. Group leaders can play a role in helping the group recognize, acknowledge, and keep in perspective the strong emotions and themes.

The group leaders must be in a place in their lives where they have come to terms with or placed in perspective the thoughts and feelings they have had related to their own distressing experience or life event. Being in the group setting with others in distress can potentially trigger difficult emotions. The group leaders need to be able to recognize and manage these situations without adding emotional burden to vulnerable group members. The goal for the self-help leaders is to initiate the group or start them on a path to expressing and operating independently or without facilitation.

Managing self-help sessions

Sessions may be started by having participants share their name (usually first name only for the sake of privacy) and their reason for coming to the group. Group "rules" should be mentioned so that members have an idea about what is expected from them and from others. It should be emphasized that the purpose of outlining rules is not to be controlling, but to create an environment where respect and expectations are equal for all. Again, self-help groups are flexible – people may attend when they want and as many sessions as they want. Self-help groups are usually open to all with a similar experience and ongoing. It should be clear what time the group starts and ends, how often the group meets, and where the group is to be held regularly (i.e. the usual location). Asking group members to respect one another's privacy is important (i.e. do not share members information with people not involved in the group). Also, the leaders should emphasize that violence of any kind (e.g. physical assault or verbal attack) is not acceptable and grounds for dismissal from the group.

The participants should be encouraged to share the actual experiences that have caused distress, how these experiences have impacted their lives and function, and the emotions they have felt as a result. The point of the group is to have members realize that they are not alone and that it is human and natural to experience emotions that can feel negative or painful. The group discussions should also help people develop an awareness of their own strengths and serve as an environment where they are constantly reminded of their strengths. In addition, hearing about ways that others have coped can help individuals increase and enhance their own methods of coping.

When individuals express strong emotions, such as anger, allow them to express openly. Their feelings should be acknowledged.

Others who can relate to the individual's emotions should share these feelings. In addition, people should be allowed to express their feelings about seeing another express anger. Allowing group members to talk about how they have managed this emotion is important. The methods mentioned by the group that have led to a sense of hope and peace should be emphasized. If there is excessive aggression or potential for abuse – remind the entire group members of the ground rules about violence and aggression.

After a number of sessions (the actual number will vary from group to group) members should have developed an idea about the purpose, structure, and operation of the group. The goal for co-leaders is to transfer this understanding, withdraw ultimately as facilitators, and allow the group to run independently.

Family Support

Family members are often the caretakers of individuals with mental conditions. They may provide the emotional and physical support and may also manage the economic expenses related to mental health treatments and care. Being exposed to distress, family members are vulnerable to becoming distressed. In addition, they may become victims of stigma by association - they may be rejected by others in the community who do not understand mental conditions, leading to a feeling of isolation and limited social activity.

Providing families with specific information and practical methods of support is important. Teaching family members about signs and symptoms of a condition, treatments, and what to expect (or not expect) from treatments is necessary. Providing advice on how to structure time and their living environments to reduce stress is helpful. Family members may find it useful to meet with a group of others who share the same situation as a means for emotional support.

Questions Families Commonly Ask:

1. Will he/she recover?

2. Can he/she work?

3. Can he/she live at home?

4. Will he/she have to take medications for life?

5. Can he/she have children?

6. (In conflict and disaster situations) Will this experience (loss, disaster, stressful event) make him/her mentally ill?

The answers to these questions may come from varied clinicians. It is important that the healthcare provider (whether it is a nurse, doctor, or mental health aide) do his or her best to address the questions directly or refer the family to the appropriate resources and providers who can address the questions.

Community Education

Community education & the stigma of mental illness

People who are different from the norm within a society may experience stigma by others who feel uneasy, embarrassed, or too threatened to talk about behavior they perceive as different. Feelings of shame, disgrace, or rejection can occur in those who are stigmatized.

The stigma surrounding mental illness is strong, has placed a wall of silence around the issue, and can be attributed to misbelief about mental conditions, misconceptions about psychiatric medications, and poor tolerance of the community of people with mental illness. Stigma towards people with a mental illness can have a detrimental effect on their ability to obtain services, their recovery, the type of treatment and support they receive, and their acceptance in the community.

Reducing stigma means empowering those with mental conditions and changing the attitudes of uninformed people in the community. It is important to highlight the individual's positive aspects and his or her capacity to make contributions to the family and society. Encourage the person to take part in the community.

A counselor can be a good model for the community by treating those suffering from mental conditions with empathy, humanity, dignity, and respect and relating to the person, not the illness. Modeling or demonstrating positive communication skills towards the individual when other people are present is a way to teach others how to interact appropriately and respectfully.

Liaising and building up trusting relationships with the families of those affected, fosters understanding and decreases frustration. Lastly, organizing activities or talks within the community to raise awareness about mental health, illness, and stigma can improve knowledge and tolerance.

Community Psychosocial Development Through Psychosocial Activities

Communities impacted by significant social stressors (e.g. chronic poverty, social/political conflict, armed conflict, natural disaster) can benefit from interventions aimed to stabilize, maintain, or develop the community's social structure and function. A community's social state is influenced by the psychological and social well-being of its members. Community psychosocial development involves helping communities organize activities, events, and projects (that members in engage in as a group) to foster social or relational well-being between individuals and psychological well-being within individuals. Psychosocial activities, events, and projects may serve as the modes or venues to bring members together to understand the facts, identify relevant issues, and devise effective solutions related to significant social stressors. Good psychosocial development of the community depends on the active participation of community members in identifying their priorities and deciding on solutions.

Purpose of psychosocial activities, events, & projects

For communities impacted by significant social stressors, psychosocial activities, events, and projects may play a role in:

1) Reestablishing a sense of normalcy;

2) Rebuilding social ties between individuals and reestablishing functioning social networks;

3) Helping community members gain knowledge and place in perspective the facts associated with the significant social stressors;

4) Helping community members identify the relevant, priority problems and issues related to the social stressor;

5) Helping the community develop effective, culture-appropriate interventions to manage the problems and issues;

6) Helping members identify and institute culture-appropriate means for generally empowering or increasing the capacity to affect their circumstances, enrich their individual lives, and enrich the structure and function of their communities.

Helping communities organize psychosocial activities, events, & projects

The process of organizing psychosocial activities, events, and projects should stem from the community and will vary from one cultural group to another. Outlined below are a few suggestions on how to facilitate the organizational process:

1. Meet with community members or representatives to assess the interest and desire for psychosocial activities, events, or projects.

2. Provide information on the purpose and potential benefits of organizing psychosocial activities, events, and projects.

3. Identify and collaborate with existing groups, organizations, or individuals who have been playing a role already in addressing the social stressors and organizing supportive activities.

4. Support and respect community members' participation in identifying their priorities and determining solutions considered effective.

Examples of psychosocial activities, events, & projects fostering community psychosocial development

A variety of modes or venues may be used to foster support and psychosocial development in communities affected by significant social stressors. Modes or venues have included recreational, cultural, educational, and work-related activities (events and projects) that are didactic and creative in nature. Listed below are a few examples:

1. Recreational activities (e.g. sports, games, hobbies).

2. Cultural events (e.g. musical concerts and other artistic performances; art exhibits).

3. Educational projects (e.g. lectures; mobile libraries; academic school quizzes/competitions).

4. Work-related projects (e.g. job training seminars; development of business organizations and networks).

MEDICATION GUIDE

The guide is intended for use by authorized prescribers only. Medications included in this section are mainly from lists of essential psychotropic medicines recommended by the World Health Organization (WHO) for use in settings where mental health care is limited or nonexistent.

General prescribing principles

1. Prior to prescribing medication be clear about the psychiatric diagnosis and target symptoms.

2. Be aware of underlying medical conditions, alcohol & drug abuse, or drug-drug interactions that may be a factor in the presenting psychiatric symptoms.

3. Be clear about expected side effects, potential drug interactions and potential for dependence.

4. Ask patients about other medications they are taking including self prescribed or herbal remedies and caution them against combining medications or consulting other practitioners without informing the prescriber.

5. Pursue full medication trials with adequate doses and duration of treatment.

6. Monitor side effects.

7. Make efforts to simplify medication regimens to encourage compliance.

8. Avoid poly-pharmacy (multiple or redundant medications).

9. Adjust doses appropriately for special populations such as the elderly and children.

10. Keep records of patient response & side effects throughout the treatment course.

Psychotropic Medications Included on WHO Model List of Essential Medicines (2011)

Medication for Psychotic Conditions

1. Chlorpromazine (hydrochloride) *(100mg tab; 25mg/5ml syrup; 25mg/ml injection in 2ml ampoule)*

2. Fluphenazine (decanoate or enantate) *(25mg in 2ml ampoule injection*)

3. Haloperidol *(2mg tab, 5mg tab; 5mg in 1ml ampoule injection)*

Medication for Depression

1. Amitriptyline (hydrochloride) *(25mg tab)*

2. Fluoxetine (20mg tabs)

Medication for Bipolar Disorder

1. Carbamazapine *(100mg scored tab; 200mg scored tab)*

2. Lithium carbonate *(300mg tab or capsule)*

3. Valproic acid *(200mg, 500mg [sodium salt] enteric coated tabs)*

Medication for Generalized Anxiety and Insomnia

1. Diazepam *(2mg, 5mg scored tab)*

Medication for Obsessive Compulsive Disorder

1. Clomipramine *(10mg, 25mg capsules)*

Medications Used in Established Substance Dependence Programs

1. Methadone *(5mg/ml, 10mg/5ml oral solutions; 5mg/ml, 10mg/ml oral solutions [hydrochloride])*

III: Conditions & Issues: Medication Guide

Medication Therapy for Schizophrenia/Psychotic Conditions

DRUG NAME	DOSING	SIDE EFFECTS	COMMENT
Chlorpromazine	Oral:10mg tid –qid or 25mg bid-tid. After 1-2 days may increase by 20-50mg twice **weekly**. Usual dose is 200-600mg daily in divided doses. Maximum dose is 800mg daily in divided doses. IM (for acute agitated psychosis): 25mg & may repeat 25mg-50mg in1-4 hours if needed. May then gradually increase by 25-50mg q 4 -6 hours. Maximum: 400-500mg / day	Sedation; constipation; urinary retention; orthostasis; arrhythmia; may make a seizure more possible in patients with an existing seizure disorder; tardive dyskinesia with long-term use	Low potential for EPS; may also be used in low dose for **agitation** not responsive to anti-anxiety medications

Drugs in the shaded boxes are included on the WHO (World Health Organization) Model List of Essential Medicines (2011).

**Atypical antipsychotic—this class is associated with the metabolic syndrome and increased mortality in elderly patients with dementia-related psychosis.*

Only common side effects are noted. Prescribers should check the medication literature for all potential side effects and drug interactions.

Children, the elderly, adults with small body composition, and individuals with medical illness or nutritional deficiencies may require smaller initial & maintenance doses for effect and may be more susceptible to side effects.

For an explanation of the abbreviations included in the tables, see the "Medical Abbreviations List" in the front of the manual.

III: Conditions & Issues: Medication Guide

(Medication therapy for schizophrenia/psychotic conditions continued…)

DRUG NAME	DOSING	SIDE EFFECTS	COMMENT
Fluphenazine (oral)	Starting dose: 2.5mg-10mg/day in divided doses at 6—8 hour intervals. May increase to a maximum 40mg/day in divided doses if necessary. Maintenance dose: 1-5mg/day.	Sedation; EPS; Tardive dyskinesia with long-term use	High potential for EPS. Not indicated for use in children.
Fluphenazine Decanoate (25mg/ml IM long-acting injection)	Initial: 12.5-25mg q 2-4 weeks. Dose may be titrated as high as 50mg IM q 2 - 4 weeks. NOTE: 12.5mg of decanoate q 2-4 weeks=10mg / day of oral	Sedation; EPS; Tardive dyskinesia with long-term use	High potential for EPS; consider use in patients with chronic psychosis who are noncompliant with oral medications. Not indicated for use in children.
Haloperidol (oral tablets & IM 5mg/ml short-acting injection as lactate)	Oral: 0.5-5mg 2-3 times/day. Maximum: 30mg/day. IM injection (lactate) for immediate tranquilization of severe agitation: 5mg q 30-60 minutes to a maximum 10-20mg.	Sedation; EPS; Tardive dyskinesia with long-term use	High potential for EPS; may also be used in low dose for **severe agitation** not responsive to anti-anxiety medications
Haloperidol Decanoate (50mg/ml long-acting injection)	Initial: 10-20 times daily oral dose q 4 weeks. Maintenance dose is 10-15 times initial oral dose. NOTE: 100mg of decanoate q 4 weeks=10mg/day of oral.	Sedation; EPS; Tardive dyskinesia with long-term use	High potential for EPS; consider use in patients with chronic psychosis who are non-compliant with oral medication. Not indicated for use in children.

*Drugs in the shaded boxes are included on the WHO Model List of Essential Medicines (2011). Only common side effects are noted. Prescribers should check the medication literature for all potential side effects and drug interactions. Children, the elderly, adults with small body composition, and individuals with medical illness or nutritional deficiencies may require smaller initial & maintenance doses for effect and may be more susceptible to side effects. For an explanation of the abbreviations included in the tables, see the "Medical Abbreviations List" in the front of the manual.

(Medication therapy for schizophrenia/psychotic conditions continued…)

DRUG NAME	DOSING	SIDE EFFECTS	COMMENT
Perphenazine	Less severe symptoms: 4-8mg, 3 times/day (Maximum: 24 mg/day) Severe symptoms: 8-16mg 2-4 times/day (maximum: 64mg/day).	Sedation; dry mouth; tachycardia; hypotension; moderate EPS; seizure	Moderate potential for EPS
**Risperidone (oral)	Initial: 2mg/day in 1-2 divided doses; may be increased by 1-2mg/day up to a maximum 6mg/day in divided doses.	Sedation; EPS; Tardive dyskinesia with long-term use	Less potential for EPS than haloperidol but EPS risk increased at doses > 4mg daily

*Drugs in the shaded boxes are included on the WHO Model List of Essential Medicines (2011).

**Atypical antipsychotic—this class is associated with the metabolic syndrome and increased mortality in elderly patients with dementia-related psychosis.

Only common side effects are noted. Prescribers should check the medication literature for all potential side effects and drug interactions.

Children, the elderly, adults with small body composition, and individuals with medical illness or nutritional deficiencies may require smaller initial & maintenance doses for effect and may be more susceptible to side effects.

For an explanation of the abbreviations included in the tables, see the "Medical Abbreviations List" in the front of the manual.

While medications from the WHO Model List of Essential
Medicines (in addition to a few drugs with different properties) have been presented previously, several other antipsychotic medications have been developed and utilized for the
treatment of psychotic conditions (e.g. schizophrenia). These
medications are listed in the table below.

Other Antipsychotic Medications

Medica-tion Class	Typical (low potency)	Typical (high potency)	Atypical
Drug Name	Prochlor-perazine Trifluop-erazine	Droperidol Loxapine Pimozide Thiothix-ene	Aripiprazole Asenapine Clozapine Iloperidone Lurasidone Olanzapine Paliperidone Quetiapine Ziprasidone

---
III: Conditions & Issues: Medication Guide

Special notes regarding antipsychotic medications

1) Remission of chronic, severe psychotic symptoms may require at least 4-6 weeks of antipsychotic medication therapy.

2) EPS = extra-pyramidal symptoms (tremor; akathisia or a subjective sense of physical restlessness; muscular stiffness or "cogwheel" rigidity; shuffling walking pattern; stooped posture; drooling or uncontrolled seepage of saliva from the mouth). Observation (e.g. viewing for tremors, drooling, stooped posture, and a shuffling walking pattern) and physical examination (e.g. flexing the elbow joints and feeling the arm muscles for tightness or rigidity) are ways to detect symptoms. Studies (western research) indicate that EPS is more common with high potency typical antipsychotics (e.g. haloperidol and fluphenazine) than with low potency antipsychotics (e.g. phenothiazines such as chlorpromazine). High doses of antipsychotic medication are associated with an increased risk for EPS. Western studies (United States) have found that symptoms are more common in men under the age of 35 who have muscular body types. EPS typically occur within the first 4 weeks of antipsychotic use and are reversible with discontinuation of the drug. Symptoms may disappear within days to months after antipsychotic medication has been stopped. If a patient needs to remain on medication to control severe psychotic symptoms, EPS may be reduced with anticholinergic medicines such as trihexyphenidyl or diphenhydramine and, for akathisia specifically, propanolol and benzodiazepines (i.e. diazepam, lorazepam, and clonazepam).

3) Tardive dyskinesia = involuntary, jerking or twisting motion of muscles (usually head, limbs, or trunk); Tardive dyskinesia is irre-versible and antipsychotic medication should be immediately dis-continued if symptoms occur.

4) Neuroleptic malignant syndrome (NMS) = can occur due to antipsychotic medication especially in those with underlying medi-cal illness. Symptoms include muscle rigidity; inability to move; mutism; unstable blood pressure or heart rate; extremely high tem-perature; sweating & agitation. This condition is life-threatening therefore medication must be discontinued immediately and emer-gent medical assistance must be sought.

5) Metabolic Syndrome = abnormalities in glucose metabolism, lipid metabolism, body weight/fat distribution, and blood pressure generally associated with schizophrenia and atypical antipsychotic medications. Patients treated with atypical antipsychotics should be monitored for these conditions.

III: Conditions & Issues: Medication Guide

Drugs to treat extra-pyramidal symptoms caused by antipsychotic medications

DRUG NAME	DOSING	SIDE EFFECTS & CONTRAINDICATIONS
Amantadine	100mg po twice daily; may increase to a maximum 300mg daily in divided doses if necessary.	Nausea; headache; orthostasis; insomnia; ataxia; anxiety; depression; hallucinations; delirium
Benztropine	1-2mg po bid – tid depending on severity of EPS. When EPS remits discontinue.	Dry mouth; constipation; blurred vision; urinary retention; hyperthermia; euphoria; delirium
Biperiden	2mg po daily—2mg po tid	Blurred vision; bradycardia; constipation; disorientation; drowsiness; dry mouth; euphoria; hypotension; orthostatic hypotension; sleep disturbance; urinary retention
Diphenhydramine	25-100mg po daily; may be increased by 25-50mg daily to 100mg/day	Sedation; dry mouth
Trihexyphenidyl	1mg po daily; safe to increase dose to up to 5-15mg/day in 3-4 divided doses.	Dry mouth; constipation; blurred vision; urinary retention; hyperthermia; euphoria; delirium

Only common side effects are noted. Prescribers should check the medication literature for all potential side effects and drug interactions. Children, the elderly, adults with small body composition, and individuals with medical illness or nutritional deficiencies may require smaller initial & maintenance doses for effect and may be more susceptible to side effects. For an explanation of the abbreviations included in the tables, see the "Medical Abbreviations List" in the front of the manual. Drugs in the shaded boxes are included on the WHO Model List of Essential Medicines (2011).

Medication Therapy For Depression

Antidepressant medications

Varied classes of antidepressant medication have been shown to be effective for symptoms of depression. Each class acts differently on neuro-chemical receptors (e.g. serotonin, norepinephrine, dopamine) in the brain to yield effects. The classes of antidepressant medications commonly used include:

Alpha-2 antagonists (atypical)

Dopamine reuptake inhibitors (atypical)

MAOI (monoamine oxidase inhibitors)

SNRI (selective norepinephrine reuptake inhibitors)

SSRI (selective serotonin reuptake inhibitor)

Tetracyclics (act on varied receptors)

Tricyclics (act on varied receptors)

SSRI, SNRI, and atypicals are newer than tetracyclic and tricyclic antidepressants and are associated with fewer side effects and less lethality if taken in overdose.

III: Conditions & Issues: Medication Guide

NOTES FOR ALL ANTIDEPRESSANT MEDICATIONS LISTED IN THIS SECTION:

1) Only common side effects are noted. Prescribers should check the medication literature for all potential side effects and drug interactions. 2) Children, the elderly, adults with small body composition, and individuals with medical illness or nutritional deficiencies may require smaller initial & maintenance doses for effect and may be more susceptible to side effects. 3) Studies in the United States have indicated that antidepressants may <u>*increase the risk of suicidal thoughts and behavior in children, adolescents, and young adults age 18-24*</u> *with major depressive disorder. A number of agents are not approved in the United States for use in the pediatric population. 4) For an explanation of the abbreviations included in the tables, see the "Medical Abbreviations List" in the front of the manual. Drugs in the shaded boxes are included on the WHO Model List of Essential Medicines (2011).*

Antidepressant Medication	DOSING	SIDE EFFECTS	COMMENT
AMITRIPTYLINE (tricyclic) *blood level monitoring is required*	50—150mg/day either as a single dose or in divided doses. May be gradually increased up to 300mg/day (divided doses). Check blood level every 1-4 weeks; *If blood test is not available, monitor for symptoms of toxicity and adjust accordingly.* Requires therapeutic blood level monitoring. Therapeutic blood level should be between 100-250ng/ml)	Sedation; arrhythmia; constipation; urinary retention; may make a seizure more possible in patients with an existing seizure disorder	*If blood test is not available, monitor for symptoms of toxicity (flu; fever; muscle/joint aches; nausea or vomiting abnormal HR; delirium)*

213

(Antidepressant medications continued...)

Antidepressant	DOSING	EFFECTIVE - MAXIMUM DOSE RANGE	SIDE EFFECTS	COMMENT
BUPROPION (dopamine-reuptake inhibitor)	Immediate Release (IR): 100mg bid; after 4 days can increase to 100mg tid. Sustained Release (SR):150mg qam for 4 days then 150mg q am & q afternoon. Extended Release (XL)=150 mg/day for 4 days then increase to 300mg/day.	IR= 300-450mg (divided doses) SR =300 - 400mg/day (divided doses) XL = 300 - 450 mg /day	seizure risk is increased with history of bulimia	*May be especially useful for depression that includes poor energy as a symptom due to its activating potential*
FLUOXETINE (SSRI)	20mg every morning (due to stimulating effect); Lower doses of 5-10mg/day have been used as a starting dose. May increase after several weeks (by 20mg/day increments. Doses>20mg/day may be given in bid doses (i.e. morning & afternoon) or as a single morning dose.	20-80mg Daily	Insomnia or agitation due to stimulating effect	*May be especially useful for depression that includes poor energy as a symptom due to its activating potential*
SERTRALINE (SSRI)	25-50mg daily; safe to increase dose by 25-50mg every 7 days to 100mg.	50-200mg daily	Gastrointestinal distress; delayed ejaculation	

While medications from the WHO Model List of Essential Medicines (in addition to a few drugs with different properties) have been presented previously, there are several other antidepressant medications that have been developed and utilized for the treatment of major depression. These medications are listed in the table below.

Other Antidepressant Medications

Medication Class	Drug Name
Alpha-2 Antagonist	Mirtazapine
Monoamine oxidase Inhibitor (MAOI)	Phenelzine selegiline Tranlcypromine
Selective Serotonin Reuptake Inhibitor (SSRI)	Citalopram Escitalopram Fluvoxamine Paroxetine Vilazodone (5HT1A partial agonist)
Serotonin/Norepinephrine Reuptake Inhibitor (SNRI)	Desvenlafaxine Duloxetine Venlafaxine
Tetracyclic	Maprotiline
Tricyclic	Amoxapine Clomipramine Desipramine Doxepin Imipramine Nortriptyline Protriptyline

Medication Therapy for Mania/Bipolar Disorder

Lithium, anticonvulsants (e.g. carbamezapine, lamotrigine, oxcar-
bazepine, topiramate, valproate) and atypical antipsychotic medications (e.g. aripiprazole, olanzapine, risperidone, ziprasidone)
have been used to manage manic symptoms. A combination of an
antidepressant (to stabilize depressive symptoms) and an anti-
manic medication (to stabilize manic symptoms) may be used con-
comitantly for treatment of bipolar disorder. An anti-psychotic
medication may be added if psychotic symptoms are present.

Medications for bipolar disorder

DRUG NAME	DOSING	SIDE EFFECTS	IINDICATION & COMMENTS
Carbamazepine

(blood level monitoring is required) | Tablets/capsules: 400mg/day in divided doses (e.g. 200mg tabs bid). Oral suspension: 400mg/day in 4 divided doses (e.g. 100mg qid). May adjust by 200mg/day increments. Maximum dose = 1600mg/day. Monitor blood levels (therapeutic range = 4-12mcg/mL). | Dizziness; stomach upset; ataxia; Rarely causes liver disease or skin rash; rarely depression of red and white blood cells causing anemia/agranulocytosis/susceptibility to infections | Stabilizes manic phase of bipolar I & mixed bipolar disorder; Normally white blood cell levels are monitored but if no test available, *monitor for symptoms of **toxicity** (flu; fever; weakness; muscle/joint aches; nausea or vomiting; abnormal HR; delirium)* |

DRUG NAME	DOSING	SIDE EFFECTS	INDICATION & COMMENTS
Lithium Carbonate

(blood level monitoring is required) | For acute mania: 600mg tid to achieve effective levels of 1-1.5mEq/L; monitor levels twice weekly until stabilized. Maintenance: 300mg tid –qid to maintain serum levels of 0.6-1.2 mE/L. Then monitor levels every 1-3 months. | Thirst; increased urination; tremor; weight gain | Stabilizes manic episodes and is maintenance treatment of bipolar disorder; *If serum test is not available monitor for evidence of toxicity (ataxia; dysarthria irritability; vomiting; confusion/delirium; stupor; seizure)* |

Drugs in the shaded boxes are included on the WHO Model List of Essential Medicines (2011). Only common side effects are noted. Prescribers should check the medication literature for all potential side effects and drug interactions. Children, the elderly, adults with small body composition, and individuals with medical illness or nutritional deficiencies may require smaller initial & maintenance doses for effect and may be more susceptible to side effects. For an explanation of the abbreviations included in the tables, see the "Medical Abbreviations List" in the front of the manual.

(Medications for bipolar disorder continued)

DRUG NAME	DOSING	SIDE EFFECTS	INDICATION/ COMMENTS
**Risperidone (oral)	Initial: 2-3mg daily; may increase dose by 1mg /day to a maximum of 6mg daily.	Sedation; EPS; Tardive dyskinesia with long-term use	Stabilizes acute manic phases or mixed episodes of bipolar disorder ; Less potential for EPS than haloperidol but EPS risk increased at doses > 4mg/day
Valproic Acid (blood level monitoring is required)	750mg/day in divided doses; increase dose rapidly to desired clinical effect. Maximum dose: 60mg/kg/day. Blood level should be monitored (therapeutic level= 50-125mcg/mL).	Gastrointestinal distress; sedation; tremor; ataxia; hepatic toxicity	Stabilizes manic phases of bipolar disorder

Drugs in the shaded boxes are included on the WHO Model List of Essential Medicines (2011). Only common side effects are noted. Prescribers should check the medication literature for all potential side effects and drug interactions. Children, the elderly, adults with small body composition, and individuals with medical illness or nutritional deficiencies may require smaller initial & maintenance doses for effect and may be more susceptible to side effects. For an explanation of the abbreviations included in the tables, see the "Medical Abbreviations List" in the front of the manual.

**Atypical antipsychotic—this class is associated with the metabolic syndrome and increased mortality in elderly patients with dementia-related psychosis.*

While medications from the WHO Model List of Essential Medicines (in addition to a few drugs with different properties) have been presented previously, other anti-manic and mood-stabilizing medications have been developed and utilized for the treatment of mania and bipolar disorder. These medications are listed below.

Other Anti-manic Medications

Medication Class	Anti-manic/ Atypical Antipsychotic	Anti-manic/ Anticonvulsant
Drug Name	Asenapine Olanzapine	Divalproex

Medication Therapy for Anxiety-Related Conditions, Post-Traumatic Stress Disorder (PTSD), & Obsessive-Compulsive Disorder (OCD)

General

a) The benzodiazepine class of medication is commonly used for anxiety but caution should be used in prescribing since tolerance, dependence, and serious withdrawal may occur. Use of the benzodiazepines in short-term is usually recommended.

b) For chronic anxiety conditions (e.g. panic disorder, obsessive-compulsive disorder, generalized anxiety disorder, post-traumatic stress, social anxiety disorder) other agents such as SSRIs (selective serotonin reuptake inhibitors – e.g. fluoxetine, paroxetine, sertraline, citalopram, escitalpram), SNRIs (selective norepinephrine reuptake inhibitors – e.g. duloxetine, venlafaxine), buspirone, and tricyclics (clomipramine) have been effective.

NOTES FOR MEDICATIONS IN THIS SECTION:

1) Only common side effects are noted. Prescribers should check the medication literature for all potential side effects and drug interactions. 2) Children, the elderly, adults with small body composition, and individuals with medical illness or nutritional deficiencies may require smaller initial & maintenance doses for effect and may be more susceptible to side effects. 3) Studies in the United States have indicated that antidepressants may increase the risk of suicidal thoughts and behavior in children, adolescents, and young adults age 18-24 with major depressive disorder (DSM IV criteria). A number of agents are not approved in the United States for use in the pediatric population. 4) For an explanation of the abbreviations included in the tables, see the "Medical Abbreviations List" in the front of the manual. Drugs in the shaded boxes are included on the WHO Model List of Essential Medicines (2011).

DRUG NAME	INDICATIONS	DOSING	SIDE EFFECTS	COMMENTS
CLOMIPRAMINE	Obsessive — Compulsive Disorder (OCD)	Initial: 25mg /day; may gradually increase as tolerated over the first 2 weeks to 100mg in divided doses. Maintenance: May further increase to recommended maximum of 250mg/day; may give as a single daily dose once tolerated.	Dry mouth, constipation, nausea,, increased appetite, weight gain, dizziness, nervousness.	No addiction potential; *Studies in the United States have indicated that antidepressants may increase the risk of suicidal thoughts and behavior in children, adolescents, and young adults age 18-24 with major depressive disorder.*

III: Conditions & Issues: Medication Guide

(Medication therapy for anxiety-related conditions continued…)

DRUG NAME	INDICATIONS	DOSING	SIDE EFFECTS	COMMENTS
DIAZEPAM	Intermittent anxiety; generalized anxiety disorder (GAD)	Oral tab or IM injection: 2 –10mg 2-4 times daily as needed	Sedation; respiratory depression; delirium	Onset in 20-30minutes; Long-acting; Has addiction potential
FLUOXETINE	Obsessive compulsive disorder (OCD); Panic disorder; post—traumatic stress disorder (PTSD); social anxiety disorder	OCD: Initial: 20mg/day; may increase after many weeks to 20-60mg/day (maximum 80mg/day). Panic disorder: Initial 10mg/day; after 1 week increase to 20mg/day; after many weeks, may continue to increase if necessary (to a maximum 60mg/day). PTSD: 20mg/day; if necessary may increase after many weeks to maximum 40mg/day. Social anxiety disorder: 20mg/day; if necessary, may increase after many weeks to a maximum 40mg/day.	Insomnia or agitation due to stimulating effect	No addiction potential; *Studies in the United States have indicated that antidepressants may increase the risk of suicidal thoughts and behavior in children, adolescents, and young adults age 18-24 with major depressive disorder.*
PAROXETINE	Generalized anxiety disorder (GAD); Obsessive compulsive disorder; panic disorder (OCD); Post traumatic stress disorder (PTSD); Social anxiety disorder	Generalized anxiety disorder: start 20mg qam; may increase weekly by 10mg qam (maximum=50mg qam but >20mg/day may not have additional benefit) OCD: start 20mg qam; may increase weekly by 10mg qam to 40mg qam (maximum=60mg qam). Panic disorder: start 10mg qam; may increase weekly by 10mg qam to 40mg qam (maximum=60mg/day). PTSD: start 20mg qam; may increase weekly by 10mg qam (maximum=50mg qam but >20mg/day may not have additional benefit). Social anxiety disorder: start 20mg qam; may increase weekly by 10mg qam (maximum=60mg qam but >20mg/day may not have additional benefit). For all disorders reduce gradually upon discontinuation.	Agitation if discontinued abruptly; gastrointestinal distress; delayed ejaculation	No addiction potential; *Studies in the United States have indicated that antidepressants may increase the risk of suicidal thoughts and behavior in children, adolescents, and young adults age 18-24 with major depressive disorder.*

Medication Therapy for Epilepsy

DRUG NAME	DOSING	SIDE EFFECTS	INDICATION & COMMENTS
Carbamazepine (blood level monitoring is required)	Initial (tablets): 400mg/day in 2 divided doses. Increase by up to 200mg/day in 3-4 divided doses until optimal response and therapeutic levels are achieved. Usual dose = 800-1200mg/day. Maximum dose = 1600mg/day. Therapeutic serum level = 4-12 mcg/mL.	dizziness; stomach upset; Rarely causes liver disease or skin rash; rarely depression of red and white blood cells causing anemia or susceptibility to infections; Normally white blood cell levels are monitored but if no test available, monitor for symptoms of **toxicity** (flu; fever; weakness; muscle/ joint aches; nausea or vomiting; abnormal HR; delirium)	Tonic-Clonic; partial (focal)
Clonazepam	Initial daily dose not to exceed 1.5mg given in 3 divided doses; may increase by 0.5-1mg every 3rd day until seizures are controlled or side effects observed. Maintenance: 0.05-0.2mg/kg; do not exceed 20mg/day.	Sedation; ataxia; confusion; respiratory depression	For absence seizure, myoclonic seizures, infantile spasms, & childhood epilepsies. There is addiction potential with this drug.
Diazepam (Rectal gel)	Acute anticonvulsant treatment: 0.2mg/kg; may be repeated in 4-12 hours if needed. Do not use for more than 5 episodes per month or more than 1 episode every 5 days.		Acute anticonvulsant treatment

NOTES: 1) Only common side effects are noted. Prescribers should check the medication literature for all potential side effects and drug interactions. 2) Children, the elderly, adults with small body composition, and individuals with medical illness or nutritional deficiencies may require smaller initial & maintenance doses for effect and may be more susceptible to side effects. 3) For an explanation of the abbreviations included in the table, see the "Medical Abbreviations List" in the front of the manual. 4) Drugs in the shaded boxes are included on the WHO Model List of Essential Medicines (2011).

(Medication Therapy for Epilepsy continued...)

DRUG NAME	DOSING	SIDE EFFECTS	INDICATION & COMMENTS
Phenobarbitol (blood level monitoring is required)	60-180mg daily. Therapeutic range = 10-40mcg/mL	Sedation; ataxia; confusion; dizziness; depression; skin rash	Tonic-clonic; partial (focal); has addiction potential
Phenytoin (blood level monitoring is required)	Initial: 100mg tid. May increase at 7-10 day intervals. Maximum: 200mg tid. Therapeutic blood level = 10-20mcg/mL	Potential toxicity; Normally blood levels are monitored due to toxicity potential but if no test available, monitor for symptoms of **toxicity** (flu; fever; weakness; muscle/joint aches; nausea or vomiting; abnormal HR; delirium)	Tonic-clonic; complex partial (focal)
Valproic Acid (blood level monitoring is required)	**Absence:** 15mg/kg/day; increase 5-10mg/kg/day at weekly intervals until therapeutic level reached. Max=60mg/kg/day. **Complex partial:** 10-15mg/kg/day, increase 5-10mg/kg/day at weekly intervals until therapeutic level reached. Max=60mg/kg/day. *Therapeutic blood level = 50-125mcg/mL*	Sedation; gastrointestinal distress; tremor; hepatic toxicity	Absence seizures; complex partial (focal); also myoclonic seizure

NOTES: 1) Only common side effects are noted. Prescribers should check the medication literature for all potential side effects and drug interactions. 2) Children, the elderly, adults with small body composition, and individuals with medical illness or nutritional deficiencies may require smaller initial & maintenance doses for effect and may be more susceptible to side effects. 3) For an explanation of the abbreviations included in the table, see the "Medical Abbreviations List" in the front of the manual. 4) Drugs in the shaded boxes are included on the WHO Model List of Essential Medicines (revised March 2011).

Medication Therapy For Sleep Disturbance

1) Every effort to correct a sleep disturbance utilizing good sleep hygiene should be attempted first prior to prescribing sedative medication. Secondary conditions contributing to the sleep disturbance need to be addressed and stabilized prior to prescribing medication.

2) See the table on the following page for specific medications that can be helpful for insomnia. In general, non-habit forming (non-addictive) medications should be tried first and medications should be prescribed in limited quantities on a prn or "as needed" basis.

III: Conditions & Issues: Medication Guide

Medications for Sleep Disturbance

SLEEP MEDICATION	DOSING	SIDE EFFECTS	COMMENT
DIAZEPAM	2-10mg at bedtime as needed.	Sedation; respiratory depression; delirium	Onset in 20-30 minutes; Long-acting; Has addiction potential
DIPHENHYDRAMINE	50mg at bedtime as needed.	Sedation; dry mouth	**No addiction potential**
LORAZEPAM	1-2mg at bedtime as needed. Maximum = 4mg at bedtime.	Sedation; respiratory depression; delirium	Onset in 20-30 minutes; short-acting; Has addiction potential
TRAZODONE	25-50mg at bedtime. Maximum = 200mg at bedtime.	Sedation; arrhythmia; constipation; urinary retention	**No addiction potential**

NOTES: 1) Only common side effects are noted. Prescribers should check the medication literature for all potential side effects and drug interactions. 2) Children, the elderly, adults with small body composition, and individuals with medical illness or nutritional deficiencies may require smaller initial & maintenance doses for effect and may be more susceptible to side effects. 3) For an explanation of the abbreviations included in the table, see the "Medical Abbreviations List" in the front of the manual. 4) Drugs in the shaded boxes are included on the WHO Model List of Essential Medicines (2011).

Medications For Agitation: Benzodiazepines

NOTES:
1) Only common side effects are noted. Prescribers should check the medication literature for all potential side effects and drug interactions. 2) Children, the elderly, adults with small body composition, and individuals with medical illness or nutritional deficiencies may require smaller initial & maintenance doses for effect and may be more susceptible to side effects. 3) For an explanation of the abbreviations included in the table, see the "Medical Abbreviations List" in the front of the manual. 4) Drugs in the shaded boxes are included on the WHO Model List of Essential Medicines (2011).

DRUG NAME	DOSING	SIDE EFFECTS	COMMENT
DIAZEPAM	Oral: 5-10mg q 30-60 minutes until effective. Maximum=40mg/day. IM (moderate agitation): 2-5mg and may repeat if needed in 3-4 hours. IM (severe): 5-10mg and may repeat if needed in 3-4 hours.	Sedation; respiratory depression; delirium	Onset in 20-30minutes; Long-acting; Has addiction potential
LORAZEPAM	Oral or IM: 1-2mg q 30-60 minutes as needed to achieve calm. Maximum: 4mg/day.	Sedation; respiratory depression; delirium	Onset in 20-30 minutes; short-acting; Has addiction potential

226

Medications For Severe Agitation: Low Dose Antipsychotics

NOTES: 1) Only common side effects are noted. Prescribers should check the medication literature for all potential side effects and drug interactions; 2) Children, the elderly, adults with small body composition, and individuals with medical illness or nutritional deficiencies may require smaller initial & maintenance doses for effect and may be more susceptible to side effects. 3) For an explanation of the abbreviations included in the table, see the "Medical Abbreviations List" in the front of the manual. 4) Drugs in the shaded boxes are included on the WHO Model List of Essential Medicines (2011).

DRUG NAME	DOSING	SIDE EFFECTS	COMMENT
Chlorpromazine (oral or IM Injection) **FOR SEVERE, ACUTE AGITATION that is <u>not</u> responsive to other anti-anxiety medications**	Oral: 25mg tid. IM: 25mg & may repeat 25mg-50mg in1-4 hours if needed. May then gradually increase by 25-50mg q 4-6 hours. Maximum: 400-500mg /day	Sedation; constipation; urinary retention; orthostasis; arrhythmia; May make a seizure more possible in patients with an existing seizure disorder; Tardive dyskinesia with long-term use	Low potential for EPS
Haloperidol (oral or IM) *FOR SEVERE, ACUTE AGITA-TION that is <u>not responsive</u> to other anti-anxiety medications*	Oral: 0.5-5mg 2-3 times/day. Maximum: 30mg/day. IM injection (lactate) for immediate tranquilization of severe agitation: 5mg q 30-60 minutes to a maximum 10-20mg.	Sedation; EPS; Tardive dyskinesia with long-term use	High potential for EPS

References

PART I: Mental Health Worldwide

Ghodse H. *International Perspectives on Mental Health*. London: Royal College of Psychiatrists; 2011. <http://public.eblib.com/ EBLPublic/PublicView.do?ptiID=730210>. Accessed August 8, 2013.

Kessler RC, Ustun TB. *The WHO World Mental Health Surveys: Global Perspectives on the Epidemiology of Mental Disorders*. New York, NY: Cambridge University Press; 2008.

Keyes, Corey L. M. *Mental Well-Being International Contributions to the Study of Positive Mental Health*. Dordrecht: Springer, 2013. <http://dx.doi.org/10.1007/978-94-007-5195-8>. Accessed August 7, 2013.

Khandelwal S, et al. Mental and Neurological Health Research Priorities Setting in Developing Countries. *Social Psychiatry and Psychiatric Epidemiology*. 2010;45(4): 487-95.

Kleinman A. Global mental health: a failure of humanity. *Lancet*. 2009;374:603–14.

Koplan JP, Bond TC, Merson MH, et al. Towards a common definition of global health. *Lancet*. 2009;373:1993–5.

Lim SS, Vos T, Flaxman AD, et al. A comparative risk assessment of burden of disease and injury attributable to 67 risk factors and risk factor clusters in 21 regions, 1990—2010: a systematic analysis for the Global Burden of Disease Study 2010. *The Lancet*. 2012; 380 (9859):2224-2260.

Miller FP. *Mental Health: Cognition, Emotion, Quality of Life, Mental Disorder, Positive Psychology, Holism, Psychological Resilience, World Health Organization, History of Mental Disorders, Global Mental Health*. Beau Bassin, Mauritius: Alphascript Pub; 2009.

References

Murray CJ, et al. Disability-Adjusted Life Years (DALYs) for 291 Diseases and Injuries in 21 Regions, 1990-2010: a Systematic Analysis for the Global Burden of Disease Study 2010. *Lancet.* 2012;380(9859): 2197-223.

Patel V. *Where There is No Psychiatrist.* London, England: Royal College of Psychiatrists; 2002.

Patel V, I. H. Minas IH, Cohen A, Prince M. *Global Mental Health: Principles and Practice.* New York : Oxford University Press; 2014.

Patel V, Prince M. Global Mental Health: A New Global Health Field Comes of Age. *JAMA.* 2010;303(19):1976-1977.

Patel V, Woodward A. *Mental and Neurological Public Health: A Global Perspective.* San Diego, CA: Academic Press/Elsevier; 2010.

Prince M, Patel V, Saxena S, et al. No health without mental health. *Lancet.* 2007;370:859–77.

Saxena S, Thornicroft G, Knapp M, Whiteford H. Resources for mental health: scarcity, inequity, and ineffi-ciency. *Lancet.* 2007;370:878–89.

Sorel, Eliot. *21st Century Global Mental Health.* Boston: Jones & Bartlett Learning; 2013.

World Health Organization (WHO). *The Global burden of disease: 2004 update.* Geneva, Switzerland: WHO; 2008.

World Health Organization (WHO). *Investing in Mental Health.* Geneva, Switzerland: WHO; 2003.

References

World Health Organization (WHO). *Mental Health Atlas.* Geneva, Switzerland: WHO; 2005.

World Health Organization (WHO). *Mental Health Atlas.* Geneva, Switzerland: WHO; 2011.

World Health Organization. Sixty-fifth world health assembly. http://www.who.int/mediacentre/events/2012/wha65/journal/en/index4.html. Published May 2012. Accessed June 16, 2012.

PART II: Mental Health Capacity Building—increasing access to care through integration & collaboration

Abel WD, Richards-Henry M, Wright EG. 2011. Integrating Mental Health into Primary Care an Integrative Collaborative Primary Care Model--the Jamaican Experience. *The West Indian Medical Journal.* 2011;60(4): 483-9.

Abhinav AS, Beinecke RH. Global Mental Health Needs, Services, Barriers, and Challenges. *International Journal of Mental Health.* 2009;38(1): 14-29.

Armstrong G, Kermode M, Raja S, et al. A Mental Health Training Program for Community Health Workers in India: Impact on Knowledge and Attitudes". *International Journal of Mental Health Systems.* 2011;5(1).

Beinecke RH, Daniels AS, Peters J, Silvestri F. Guest Editors' Introduction: The International Initiative for Mental Health Leadership (IIMHL): A Model for Global Knowledge Exchange. *International Journal of Mental Health.* 2009;38(1): 3-13.

References

Bhana A, Petersen I, Baillie KL, Flisher AJ, and The Mhapp Research Programme Consortium. Implementing the World Health Report 2001 Recommendations for Integrating Mental Health into Primary Health Care: a Situation Analysis of Three African Countries: Ghana, South Africa and Uganda. *International Review of Psychiatry (Abingdon, England)*. 2010;22(6): 599-610.

Cohen NL, Galea S. *Population Mental Health Evidence, Policy, and Public Health Practice*. Abingdon, Oxon [England]: Routledge; 2011. <http://public.eblib.com/EBLPublic/PublicView.do?ptiID=684004>. Accessed August 7, 2013.

Daly J. *Training in Developing Nations: A Handbook for Expatriates*. Armonk, N.Y.: M.E. Sharpe; 2005.

Fricchione GL, Borba CP, Alem A, et al. Capacity Building in Global Mental Health: Professional Training. *Harvard Review of Psychiatry*. 2012;20(1).

Jenkins R, Mussa M, Haji SA, et al. *Developing and Implementing Mental Health Policy in Zanzibar, a Low Income Country Off the Coast of East Africa*. BioMed Central Ltd. BioMed Central Ltd; 2011. <http://www.ijmhs.com/content/5/1/6>. Accessed August 8, 2013.

Jorm AF. Mental Health Literacy: Empowering the Community to Take Action for Better Mental Health. *The American Psychologist*. 2012;67(3): 231-43.

Kauye F, Chiwandira C, Wright J. Increasing the Capacity of Health Surveillance Assistants in Community Mental Health Care in a Developing Country, Malawi. *Malawi Medical Journal : the Journal of Medical Association of Malawi*. 2011;23(3): 85-8.

References

Kiima D, Jenkins R. *Mental Health Policy in Kenya -an Integrated Approach to Scaling Up Equitable Care for Poor Populations*. BioMed Central Ltd. BioMed Central Ltd; 2010. <http://www.ijmhs.com/content/4/1/19>. Accessed August 8, 2013.

Lancet Global Mental Health Group. Scaling up services for mental disorders-a call for action. *Lancet*. 2007;370:1241–52.

Livingstone A. *Social Policy in Developing Countries*. Hoboken: Taylor & Francis; 2012. http://public.eblib.com/EBLPublic/PublicView.do?ptiID=614835. Accessed August 7, 2013.

Médecins Sans Frontières. Training. In *Mental Health Guidelines*. Amsterdam, Netherlands: MSF, 2005: 102-105.

Minas H. The Centre for International Mental Health Approach to Mental Health System Development. *Harvard Review of Psychiatry*. 2012;20(1).

Ogunnubi PO, Adikea CD, Oshodi Y,et al. 593 - Sociodemographic Profile, Presentations and Therapeutic Interventions in a Community Psychiatry Service in South-West, Nigeria. *European Psychiatry*. 2013;28: 1.

Omigbodun O. Developing Child Mental Health Services in Resource-Poor Countries. *International Review of Psychiatry (Abingdon, England)*. 2008;20(3): 225-35.

Patel V, Weiss HA, Chowdhary N, et al. Effectiveness of an intervention led by lay health counsellors for depressive and anxiety disorders in primary care in Goa, India (MANAS): A cluster randomised controlled trial. *The Lancet*. 2010; 376 (9758): pp. 2086-2095.

References

Petersen I, Lund C, Stein DJ. Optimizing Mental Health Services in Low-Income and Middle-Income Countries. *Current Opinion in Psychiatry.* 2011;24(4): 318-23.

Petersen I, Ssebunnya J, Bhana A, Baillie K, and MhaPP Research Programme Consortium. *Lessons from Case Studies of Integrating Mental Health into Primary Health Care in South Africa and Uganda.* BioMed Central Ltd. BioMed Central Ltd; 2011. <http://www.ijmhs.com/content/5/1/8>. Accessed August 8, 2013.

Rost K. Disability from depression: the public health challenge to primary care. *Nord J Psychiatry.* 2009;63(1):17-21.

Thornicroft G. *Global Mental Health: Putting Community Care into Practice.* Chichester, West Sussex: John Wiley & Sons; 2011.

Thornicroft G. *Community Mental Health Putting Policy into Practice Globally.* Oxford: Wiley-Blackwell; 2011. <http://dx.doi.org/10.1002/9781119979203>. Accessed August 7, 2013.

Thornicroft G. *Oxford Textbook of Community Mental Health.* Oxford: Oxford University Press; 2011.

Thornicroft G, Cooper S, Bortel TV, et al. Capacity Building in Global Mental Health Research". *Harvard Review of Psychiatry.* 2012;20(1).

Ubesie, Amelia. *Has implementation of integrated mental health services in primary care programs positively impacted health outcomes among the mentally ill in developing countries?* DigitalCommons@The Texas Medical Center; 2010. <http://digitalcommons.library.tmc.edu/dissertations/AAI1474736>. Accessed August 8, 2013.

References

Van Dyke C, L Tong, and K Mack. Global Mental Health Training for United States Psychiatric Residents. *Academic Psychiatry : the Journal of the American Association of Directors of Psychiatric Residency Training and the Association for Academic Psychiatry.* 2011;35(6): 354-9.

Weiss S, Haber J, Horowitz J, et al. The Inextricable Nature of Mental and Physical Health: Implications for Integrative Care. *Journal of the American Psychiatric Nurses Association.* 2009;15 (6): 371-382.

World Health Organization (WHO). *The Effectiveness of Mental Health Services in Primary Care: View from the Developing World.* Geneva, Switzerland: WHO; 2001.

World Health Organization. *Human Resources and Training in Mental Health Mental Health Policy & Services Guidance package.* [S.l.]: World Health Organization; 2005.

World Health Organization (WHO). *Mental Health Systems in Selected Low- and Middle-Income Countries A WHO-AIMS Cross-National Analysis.* Geneva, Switzerland: World Health Organization; 2009. http://public.eblib.com/EBLPublic/PublicView.do? ptiID=483474. Accessed August 7, 2013.

World Health Organization, and World Organization of National Colleges, Academies, and Academic Associations of General Practitioners/Family Physicians. *Integrating Mental Health into Primary Care: A Global Perspective.* Geneva, Switzerland: World Health Organization; 2008.

References

PART III: Mental Health Conditions & Issues: Identification & Interventions

Almond, Palo. Postnatal Depression: A Global Public Health Perspective. *Perspectives in Public Health.* 2009;129(5): 221-227.

American Psychiatric Association. *Diagnostic and Statistical Manual of Mental Disorders DSM V.* 5th ed. Washington, D. C.: American Psychiatric Association; 2013.

American Public Health Association (APHA). Adherence to HIV Treatment Regimens: Recommendations for Best Practices. http://www.apha.org/NR/rdonlyres/A030DDB1-02C8-4D80-923B-7EF6608D62F1/0/BestPracticesnew.pdf . Revised June 2004. Accessed 11/5/2012.

Andrews G, Cuijpers P, Craske MG, McEvoy P, Titov N. Computer therapy for the anxiety and depressive disorders is effective, acceptable and practical health care: a meta-analysis. *PLoS One.* 2010; Oct 13;5(10):e13196.

Baldessarini RJ. *Chemotherapy in Psychiatry Pharmacologic Basis of Treatments for Major Mental Illness.* New York, NY: Springer; 2013. <http://www.springerlink.com/openurl.asp?genre=book&isbn=978-1-4614-3709-3>.

Banerjee D. Road Traffic Noise and Self-Reported Sleep Disturbance: Results from a Cross-Sectional Study in Western India. *Noise and Vibration Worldwide.* 2013;44(2): 10-17.

Bolton P, Bass J, Neugebauer R, et al. Group interpersonal psychotherapy for depression in rural Uganda randomized controlled trial. *JAMA.* 2003;289(23):3117-3124.

References

Centers for Disease Control and Prevention. Attention-Deficit / Hyperactivity Disorder (ADHD). http://www.cdc.gov/ncbddd/ adhd/. Updated April 2013. Accessed August 1, 2013.

Centers for Disease Control and Prevention. Autism spectrum disorders (ASDs). http://www.cdc.gov/ncbddd/autism/index.html. Updated August 2012. Accessed August 1, 2013.

Centers for Disease Control and Prevention. Burden of Mental Illness. http://www.cdc.gov/mentalhealth/basics/burden.htm. Updated July 1, 2011. Accessed June 29,2013.

Centers for Disease Control and Prevention (CDC). How HIV Tests Work. CDC Web site. http://www.cdc.gov/Hiv/topics/ testing/resources/qa/tests_work.htm. Revised April 9, 2010. Accessed 11/5/2012.

Centers for Disease Control and Prevention (CDC). HIV/AIDs statistics and surveillance. CDC Web site. http://www.cdc.gov/ hiv/topics/surveillance/basic.htm#incidence. Updated April 23, 2013. Accessed May 22, 2013.

Centers for Disease Control and Prevention (CDC). The Role of STD Prevention and Treatment in HIV Prevention. CDC Web site. http:// http://www.cdc.gov/std/hiv/STDFact-STD-HIV.htm. Updated December 17, 2012. Accessed December 21, 2012.

Centers for Disease Control and Prevention. Tourette Syndrome (TS). http://www.cdc.gov/ncbddd/tourette/data.html. Updated April 2012. Accessed August 1, 2013.

Chandra PS. *Contemporary Topics in Women's Mental Health: Global Perspectives in a Changing Society*. Chichester, UK: Wiley -Blackwell; 2009.

References

Chandrashekar CR, Math SB. Psychosomatic Disorders in Developing Countries: Current Issues and Future Challenges. *Current Opinion in Psychiatry.* 2006;19(2): 201-6.

Chang A, Reid K, Gourineni R, Zee P. 2009. Sleep Timing and Circadian Phase in Delayed Sleep Phase Syndrome. *Journal of Biological Rhythms.* 2009; 24(4): 313-321.

Chisholm D, Sanderson K, Ayuso-Mateos JL, Saxena S. Reducing the global burden of depression: population-level analysis of intervention cost-effectiveness in 14 world regions. *Br J Psychiatry.* 2004 May; 184:393-403.

Chokroverty S. *100 Questions & Answers About Sleep and Sleep Disorders.* Sudbury, Mass: Jones and Bartlett Publishers; 2008.

Cohen M, Goforth H, Lux J, Batista S, Khalife S, Cozza K, Soffer J. *Handbook of AIDS Psychiatry.* New York City, New York: Oxford University Press; 2010.

Cookson, J, Katona, C, and Taylor, D. *Use of Drugs in Psychiatry.* London, England: Gaskell/The Royal College of Psychiatrists; 2002.

Cuijpers P, Beekman A, Reynolds C. Preventing Depression, A Global Priority. *JAMA.* 2012;307(10):1033-1034.

Delaney B, Scheiber D. *Surviving the Shadows A Journey of Hope into Post-Traumatic Stress.* Naperville, Ill: Sourcebooks; 2011. <http://public.eblib.com/EBLPublic/PublicView.do?ptiID=737051>. Accessed August 8, 2013.

Department of Health and Human Services. Panel on Antiretroviral Guidelines for Adults and Adolescents/Guidelines for the use of antiretroviral agents in HIV-1-infected adults and adolescents. AIDSinfo Web site. http://aidsinfo.nih.gov/guidelines. Updated February 12, 2013. Accessed May 22, 2013.

References

De Souza MA, Salum GA, Jarros RB, et al. Cognitive-Behavioral Group Therapy for Youths with Anxiety Disorders in the Community: Effectiveness in Low and Middle Income Countries. *Behavioural and Cognitive Psychotherapy*. 2013;41(3): 255-64.

Douglas, Anne. Working with bereaved asylum-seekers and refugees. *Bereavement Care*. 2010;29(3): 5-9.

Eddleston M, Davidson R, Brent A, Wilkinson R. *Oxford Handbook of Tropical Medicine*. 3rd ed. New York, NY: Oxford University Press; 2008. http://oxfordmedicine.com/view/10.1093/med/9780199204090.001.0001/med-9780199204090. Accessed August 7, 2013.

Ezard N, Van Ommeren, García-Moreno C. *Responding to the Psychosocial and Mental Health Needs of Sexual Violence Survivors in Conflict-Affected Settings, 28-30 November 2011, Park & Suites Hotel, Ferney-Voltaire, France: Final Report*. Geneva, Switzerland: World Health Organization; 2012. http://cpwg.net/wp-content/uploads/2012/03/Responding-to-the-Psychosocial-and-Mental-Health-Needs-of-Sexual-Violence-Survivors-in-Conflict-Affected-Settings-Final-Report-IA-3-March-2012.pdf.

Fisher J, Cabral de Mello M, V Patel, A Rahman, T Tran, S Holton, and W Holmes. 2012. "Prevalence and Determinants of Common Perinatal Mental Disorders in Women in Low- and Lower-Middle-Income Countries: a Systematic Review". *Bulletin of the World Health Organization*. 90, no. 2.

Fleury MJ, A Imboua, D Aubé, L Farand, and Y Lambert. General Practitioners' Management of Mental Disorders: a Rewarding Practice with Considerable Obstacles. *BMC Family Practice*. 2012;13.

Flisher AJ, Dawes A, Kafaar Z, et al. Child and Adolescent Mental Health in South Africa. *Journal of Child and Adolescent Mental Health*; 2012;24(2).

Gadelha A, Noto CS, de Jesus Mari J. Pharmacological Treatment of Schizophrenia. *International Review of Psychiatry (Abingdon, England).* 2012;24(5): 489-98.

Garralda ME, Raynaud JP. *Increasing Awareness of Child and Adolescent Mental Health.* Lanham, MD: Jason Aronson; 2010.

Girdano D, Dusek D, Everly GS. *Controlling Stress and Tension.* San Francisco: Pearson/Benjamin Cummings; 2005.

Giunta B, et al. Psychiatric Complications of HIV Infection: An Overview. *Psychiatric Annals.* 2013;43(5):199-203.

Gradisar M, Gardner G, Dohnt H. Recent Worldwide Sleep Patterns and Problems During Adolescence: a Review and Meta-Analysis of Age, Region, and Sleep. *Sleep Medicine. 2011;*12(2): 110-8.

Harris N, Baker J, Gray R. *Medicines Management in Mental Health Care.* Chichester, U.K.: Wiley-Blackwell; 2009. <http://public.eblib.com/EBLPublic/PublicView.do?ptiID=470127>. Accessed August 8, 2013.

Hays DG, Erford BT. *Developing Multicultural Counseling Competence: A Systems Approach.* Boston: Pearson; 2014.

Herrman H, Maj M, Sartorius N. *Depressive Disorders.* John Wiley & Sons; 2009. <http://www.myilibrary.com?id=218886&ref=toc>. Accessed August 8, 2013.

Hill L, Lee KC. Pharmacotherapy Considerations in Patients with HIV and Psychiatric Disorders: Focus on Antidepressants and Antipsychotics. *The Annals of Pharmacotherapy.* 2013;47(1): 75-89.

References

Hollifield M, Verbillis-Kolp S, Farmer B, et al. The Refugee Health Screener-15 (RHS-15): Development and Validation of an Instrument for Anxiety, Depression, and PTSD in Refugees. *General Hospital Psychiatry.* 2013;35(2).

Inter-Agency Standing Committee (IASC) Taskforce on Gender in Humanitarian Assistance. Guidelines for Gender-Based Violence Interventions in Humanitarian Settings: Focusing on Prevention of and Response to Sexual Violence in Emergencies. Refworld Web site. http://www.unhcr.org/refworld/docid/439474c74.html. Published September 2005. Accessed March 22, 2013.

Inter-Agency Standing Committee (IASC) Task Force on Mental Health & Psychosocial Support. *Guidelines on Mental Health and Psychosocial Support in Emergency Settings.* Geneva, Switzerland: WHO; 2007.

The Joint United Nations Programme on HIV/AIDS (UNAIDS). 2009 AIDS Epidemic Update. http://www.unaids.org/en/media/unaids/contentassets/dataimport/pub/report/2009/jc1700_epi_update_2009_en.pdf. Published November 2009. Accessed November 9, 2012.

The Joint United Nations Programme on HIV/AIDS (UNAIDS). *Global Facts and Figures.* New York, NY: UNAIDS; 2006.

Joseph J, et al. Global NeuroAIDS Roundtable. *Journal of Neurovirology.* 2013;19(1): 1-9.

Kieling C, Baker-Henningham H, Belfer M, et al. Child and adolescent mental health worldwide: Evidence for action. *The Lancet.* 2011;378(9801):1515-1525.

References

Kinser PA, Bourguignon C, Taylor AG, Steeves R. A Feeling of Connectedness": Perspectives on a Gentle Yoga Intervention for Women with Major Depression. *Issues in Mental Health Nursing.* 2013;34(6): 402-11.

Klasen H, and AC Crombag. What Works Where? A Systematic Review of Child and Adolescent Mental Health Interventions for Low and Middle Income Countries. *Social Psychiatry and Psychiatric Epidemiology.* 2013;48(4): 595-611.

Kotze E, Els L, Rajuili-Masilo N. Women ... Mourn and Men Carry on&Quot;: African Women Storying Mourning Practices--A South African Example. *Death Studies.* 2012;36(8): 742-766.

Kubler-Ross E. *On Death and Dying.* New York, NY: Simon & Schuster, Inc; 1969.

Kumar U, Mandal MK. *Suicidal Behaviour: Assessment of People-at-Risk.* New Delhi, India: Sage Publications; 2010.

Lexi-Comp, Inc. *Drug Information Handbook 2012-2013: A Comprehensive Resource for All Clinicians and Healthcare Professionals.* 21st ed. Hudson, OH: Lexicomp; 2012.

Longo D, Fauci A, Kasper D, Hauser S, Jameson J, Loscalzo J. *Harrison's Principles of Internal Medicine Manual of Medicine.* 18th Edition. USA: McGraw; 2013.

Luby JL. Treatment of Anxiety and Depression in the Preschool Period. *Journal of the American Academy of Child &Amp; Adolescent Psychiatry.* 2013;52(4): 346-358.

Marchetti-Mercer MC. Those Easily Forgotten: the Impact of Emigration on Those Left Behind. *Family Process.* 2012;51, no. 3: 376-90.

References

McNamara, Patrick. *Dementia*. Santa Barbara, Calif: Praeger; 2011.

Médecins Sans Frontières (MSF). Individual Treatment and Support. In *Mental Health Guidelines*. Amsterdam, Netherlands: MSF; 2005: 40-51.

Merikangas, KR; Jin, R; He, J; et al. Prevalence and correlates of bipolar spectrum disorder in the world mental health survey initiative. *Arch Gen Psychiatry*. 2011;68:241-251.

Mollica RF. *Textbook of Global Mental Health: Trauma and Recovery ; a Companion Guide for Field and Clinical Care of Traumatized People Worldwide*. [Cambridge, Mass.]: Harvard Program in Refugee Trauma; 2011.

Muñoz RF, Cuijpers P, Smit F, Barrera AZ, Leykin Y. Prevention of major depression. *Annu Rev Clin Psychol*. 2010;6:181–212.

National Institute of Allergy and Infectious Disease (NIAID). Classes of HIV/AIDS Antiretroviral Drugs. National Institutes of Health/NIAID Web site. http://www.niaid.nih.gov/topics/HIVAIDS/Understanding/Treatment/Pages/arvDrugClasses.aspx. Updated March 26, 2009. Accessed November 12, 2012.

National Institutes of Health (US Department of Health & Human Services). Intellectual and Developmental Disabilities. http://report.nih.gov/NIHfactsheets/ViewFactSheet.aspx?csid=100. Updated March 2013. Accessed August 1, 2013.

National Institute of Neurological Disorders and Stroke (NINDS). Neurological Complications of AIDS. National Institutes of Health/NINDS Web site. http://www.ninds.nih.gov/disorders/aids/aids.htm. Updated March 13, 2013. Accessed March 14, 2013.

References

Nock M, Borges G, Ono Y. *Suicide: Global Perspectives from the WHO World Mental Health Surveys*. Cambridge: Cambridge University Press; 2012.

Nuevo R, Chatterji S, Verdes E, et al. The Continuum of Psychotic Symptoms in the General Population: a Cross-National Study".*Schizophrenia Bulletin*. 2012;38(3): 475-85.

Ogden T, Hagen KA. *Adolescent Mental Health: Prevention and Intervention*. Hove, East Sussex : Routledge; 2014.

Olagunju A, et al. Toward the Integration of Comprehensive Mental Health Services in HIV Care: An Assessment of Psychiatric Morbidity Among HIV-Positive Individuals in Sub-Saharan Africa. *AIDS Care*. 2013;(2): 1-6.

Olfson M, He J, Merikangas K. Psychotropic Medication Treatment of Adolescents: Results From the National Comorbidity Survey-Adolescent Supplement. *Journal of the American Academy of Child &Amp; Adolescent Psychiatry*. 2013;52(4): 378-388.

Omigbodun O. Developing Child Mental Health Services in Resource-Poor Countries. *International Review of Psychiatry (Abingdon, England)*. 2008;20(3): 225-35.

Patel V, Flisher AJ, Nikapota A, Malhotra S. Promoting Child and Adolescent Mental Health in Low and Middle Income Countries. *Journal of Child Psychology and Psychiatry*. 2008;49(3): 313 -334.

Patel V, Thornicroft G. Packages of Care for Mental, Neurological, and Substance Use Disorders in Low- and Middle-Income Countries: PLoS Medicine Series. PLoS Med 2009;6(10): e1000160. doi:10.1371/journal.pmed.1000160.

References

Patterson V, Gautam N, Pant P. Training Non-Neurologists to Diagnose Epilepsy. *Seizure: European Journal of Epilepsy.* 2013;22 (4): 306-308.

Peltzer, Karl, and Supa Pengpid. *Health Behavior Interventions in Developing Countries.* New York: Nova Science Publishers; 2011.

Physician's Desk Reference (PDR) Network. *Physician's Desk Reference 2013.* 67th ed. Montvale, NJ: PDR Network; 2012.

Preedy VR, Watson RR. *Handbook of Disease Burdens and Quality of Life Measures.* New York: Springer; 2010.

Prick AE, de Lange J, Scherder E, Pot AM. *Home-Based Exercise and Support Programme for People with Dementia and Their Caregivers: Study Protocol of a Randomised Controlled Trial.* BioMed Central Ltd. BioMed Central Ltd; 2011. <http://www.biomedcentral.com/1471-2458/11/894>. Accessed August 8, 2013.

Rahman A, Patel V, Maselko J, Kirkwood B. The neglected 'm' in MCH programmes–why mental health of mothers is important for child nutrition. *Trop Med Int Health* 2008; 13: 579-83.

Rathbun C, Greenfield R. Antiretroviral Therapy for HIV Infection. Medscape Reference Web site. http://emedicine.medscape.com/article/1533218-overview. Updated September 12, 2012. Accessed November 7, 2012.

Rost K. Disability from depression: the public health challenge to primary care. *Nord J Psychiatry.* 2009; 63(1):17-21.

Royal College of Psychiatrists. Cognitive Behavioural Therapy. http://www.rcpsych.ac.uk/info/factsheets/pfaccog.asp. Updated February 2012. Accessed May 22, 2013.

References

Sadock B, Sadock V, Ruiz P. *Comprehensive Textbook of Psychiatry*. 9th ed. Philadelphia, PA: Lippincott Williams & Wilkins; 2009.

Scahill L, Bitsko RH, Visser SN, Blumberg SJ. Prevalence of Diagnosed Tourette Syndrome in Persons Aged 6—17 Years --- United States, 2007. *Morbidity and Mortality Weekly Report.* 2009;58(21):581-585. http://www.cdc.gov/mmwr/preview/mmwrhtml/mm5821a1.htm._Accessed August 1, 2013.

Sciberras E, Efron D, Schilpz EJ, et al. Vicki Anderson, Brad Jongeling, Philip Hazell, Obioha C Ukoumunne, and Jan M Nicholson. The Children€™s Attention Project: a Community-Based Longitudinal Study of Children with ADHD and Non-ADHD Controls". *BMC Psychiatry.* 2013;13(1).

Shidhaye R, Mendenhall E, Sumathipala K, et al. Association of Somatoform Disorders with Anxiety and Depression in Women in Low and Middle Income Countries: a Systematic Review. *International Review of Psychiatry (Abingdon, England).* 2013;25(1): 65-76.

Sphere Project. *The Humanitarian Charter. Humanitarian Charter and Minimum Standards in Disaster Response.* Geneva, Switzerland: Sphere Project; 2004.

Subramaniam ME. Abdin, Vaingankar JA, Chong SA. Prevalence, Correlates, Comorbidity and Severity of Bipolar Disorder: Results from the Singapore Mental Health Study. *Journal of Affective Disorders.* 2013;146(2): 189-196.

Sullivan S, Lewis G, Wiles N, Thompson A, Evans J. Psychotic Experiences and Social Functioning: a Longitudinal Study. *Social Psychiatry and Psychiatric Epidemiology.* 2013;48(7): 1053-65.

References

Taye H, Awoke T, Zewude F. P-1115 - Prevalence of Conventional Antipsychotic Induced Movement Disorders and Factors Associated with Them Among Psychotic Patients Treated at Amanuel Mental Specialized Hospital; Aa, Ethiopia. *European Psychiatry.* 2012; 27: 1.

Tol WA, Song S, Jordans M. Annual Research Review: Resilience and Mental Health in Children and Adolescents Living in Areas of Armed Conflict - a Systematic Review of Findings in Low- and Middle-Income Countries. *Journal of Child Psychology and Psychiatry.* 2013;54(4): 445-460.

Tran TD, Tran T, Fisher J. Validation of the Depression Anxiety Stress Scales (DASS) 21 As a Screening Instrument for Depression and Anxiety in a Rural Community-Based Cohort of Northern Vietnamese Women. *BMC Psychiatry.* 2013;13.

United Nations Office on Drugs and Crime (UNODC). *World Drug Report, 2012.* Vienna, Austria: United Nations Office on Drugs and Crime (UNODC); 2012.

Van Dijk MK, Verbraak MJ, Oosterbaan DB, van Balkom AJ. Implementing Practice Guidelines for Anxiety Disorders in Secondary Mental Health Care: a Case Study. *International Journal of Mental Health Systems.* 2012;6(1).

Van Dyke C. Research Policies for Schizophrenia in the Global Health Context. *International Journal of Mental Health.* 2013;42 (1): 51-76.

Van Loon A, van Schaik A, Dekker J, Beekman A. Bridging the Gap for Ethnic Minority Adult Outpatients with Depression and Anxiety Disorders by Culturally Adapted Treatments. *Journal of Affective Disorders.* 2013;147(1)-3: 1-3.

References

Van Ommeren M, Barbui C, de Jong K, Dua T, Jones L, et al. (2011) If You Could Only Choose Five Psychotropic Medicines: Updating the Interagency Emergency Health Kit. PLoS Med 8(5): e1001030. doi:10.1371/journal.pmed.1001030.

Viana MC, et al. Family Burden Related to Mental and Physical Disorders in the World: Results from the WHO World Mental Health (WMH) Surveys. *Revista Brasileira De Psiquiatria (São Paulo, Brazil : 1999).* 2013;35(2): 115-25.

Vostanis, Panos. Mental Health Services for Children in Public Care and Other Vulnerable Groups: Implications for International Collaboration. *Clinical Child Psychology and Psychiatry.* 2010;15 (4): 555-571.

Watkins, Christine. *Teen Suicide.* Detroit : Greenhaven Press; 2014.

World Health Organization (WHO). Atlas: global resources for persons with intellectual disabilities 2007. http://whqlibdoc.who.int/publications/2007/9789241563505_eng.pdf Published 2007. Accessed August 1, 2013.

World Health Organization (WHO). Epilepsy. Fact sheet N 999. http://www.who.int/mediacentre/factsheets/fs999/en/. Published October 2012. Accessed August , 1, 2013.

World Health Organization (WHO). Global HIV/AIDS response epidemic update and health sector progress towards universal access: progress report 2011. http://whqlibdoc.who.int/publications/2011/9789241502986_eng.pdf. Published 2011. Access November 9, 2012.

World Health Organization (WHO). *Global status report on alcohol and health.* Geneva, Switzerland: World Health Organization; 2011.

References

World Health Organization (WHO). *HIV/AIDS and Mental Health: Report by the Secretariat.* Geneva, Switzerland: WHO; 2008; p 1-5.

World Health Organization. How can suicide be prevented? http://www.who.int/features/qa/24/en/index.html. Published August 2012. Accessed August 1, 2013.

World Health Organization (WHO). *Interim WHO clinical staging of HIV/AIDS and HIV/AIDS case definitions for surveillance: African region.* Geneva, Switzerland: WHO; 2005.

World Health Organization (WHO). *International Classification of Mental and Behavioral Disorders: ICD - 10.* Geneva, Switzerland: WHO; 1992.

World Health Organization (WHO). Maternal mental health and child health and development in low and middle income countries: report of the meeting held in Geneva, Switzerland, 30 January - 1 February, 2008.

World Health Organization. mhGAP intervention guide for mental, neurological and substance use disorders in non-specialized health settings. http://whqlibdoc.who.int/publications/2010/9789241548069_eng.pdf. Published 2010. Accessed June 16, 2012.

World Health Organization (WHO). *Model List of Essential Medicines.* Geneva, Switzerland: WHO; 2005.

World Health Organization (WHO). Need to address mental disorders in children. http://www.who.int/mediacentre/news/releases/2009/autism_children_20090402/en/. Published April 2009. Accessed July 31, 2013.

References

World Health Organization. *Pharmacological Treatment of Mental Disorders in Primary Health Care*. Geneva: World Health Organization; 2009. <http://public.eblib.com/EBLPublic/PublicView.do?ptiID=557634>. Accessed August 8, 2013.

World Health Organization (WHO). *Some Strategies to Help Families Cope with Stress*. Pakistan: WHO; 2005.

Wycoff, Susan, Rattanaklao Tinagon, and Shannon Dickson. Therapeutic Practice With Cambodian Refugee Families: Trauma, Adaptation, Resiliency, and Wellness. *The Family Journal*. 2011;19(2): 165-173.

Yang L, Chen S, Chen CM, et al. Schizophrenia, Culture and Neuropsychology: Sensory Deficits, Language Impairments and Social Functioning in Chinese-Speaking Schizophrenia Patients. *Psychological Medicine. 2012;*42(7): 1485-94.

Zarate CA. *New insights, new directions for treating major depression and bipolar disorder*. Bethesda, Md: National Institutes of Health,; 2008. <http://videocast.nih.gov/launch.asp?14809>. Accessed August 8, 2013.

Zinck KE, Cutcliffe JR. Hope Inspiration Among People Living with HIV/AIDS: Theory and Implications for Counselors. *Journal of Mental Health Counseling*. 2013;35(1): 60-75.

Index

Index

Index

253

Index

Index

Index

Index

Index

Index